CORONARY CARE IN THE COMMUNITY

CORONARY CARE
IN THE COMMUNITY

Edited by
DR AUBREY COLLING

CROOM HELM   LONDON

© 1977 Aubrey Colling
Croom Helm Ltd, 2/10 St. John's Road, London SW11

British Library Cataloguing in Publication Data

Coronary care in the community.
  1. Coronary heart disease
  I. Colling, Aubrey
  616.1'23   RC685.C6

  ISBN 0-85664-481-1

Printed in Great Britain by Biddles Ltd, Guildford, Surrey

CONTENTS

ACKNOWLEDGEMENTS

My thanks are due to Dr John Fry who first planted the idea of bringing together those general practitioners who had a special interest in coronary care. The concept of a National Workshop grew, and was supported by the Newcastle Postgraduate Institute and the District Management Team of the North Tees General Hospital.

Professor Julian made many useful suggestions in the planning stages and played a large part in ensuring its eventual success. Dr Alex Dellipiani helped with details of the programme and together with other North Tees Hospital physicians (Dr Guy Warnock, Dr Kenneth Chalmers, Dr Fred Gibbons, Dr. Peter MacCormack, Dr David Carr) kindly spent many hours teaching electrocardiography to general practitioners.

I am grateful to the principal speakers, all of whom gave enthusiastic support and subsequently agreed to submit chapters for publication; also to those general practitioners who prepared group reports and to the many course members, some of whom travelled great distances to attend the workshop. There was scepticism about the willingness of general practitioners to work twelve hours a day for a week to study cardiology but I was pleased at the end of the course to find that my faith in them had been justified and my optimism well founded.

The final chapter on prevention proved specially difficult and I am grateful for help from Dr Turner and Dr Rankin who had worked closely together and considered many of the problems of prevention in general practice.

Mrs Noreen Caine organised the National Workshop and used her special skills to achieve what we had planned without mishap. She recorded and prepared drafts of the proceedings and later helped to assemble this book for publication. Her assistance is greatly appreciated.

My wife, Dr Edith Colling and partner, Dr Gwyn Davies very kindly and ably corrected the drafts of this book and made many helpful suggestions.

Though some form of publication of the proceedings of the workshop had always been in my mind I am grateful to Dr Geoffrey Marsh for finally encouraging me to produce it in the form of a book.

Lastly I would like to thank the following drug companies which exhibited drugs and equipment pertinent to primary coronary care at the workshop and made generous donations to our postgraduate fund:

Acknowledgements

Astra Chemicals Limited; British Oxygen Company; Cambridge Medical Instruments Limited; Cardiac Recorders Limited; Cardio Vascular Instruments Limited; Duncan, Flockhart and Company Limited; Imperial Chemical Industries; Sandoz Products Limited; Simonsen and Weel Limited; Chas. F. Thackray Limited; Vitalograph Medical Instrumentation.

INTRODUCTION

Dr Aubrey Colling

In 1975 the results of the Teesside Coronary Survey, described in Chapter 3, became available, and appeared to cast further doubts on the benefits to be gained from the practice of sending patients who had suffered a coronary thrombosis into coronary care units. Even after taking into consideration age, sex and the severity of attacks, patients appeared to do equally well, if not better, at home. Some of the pioneers of coronary care units had turned their attentions to providing earlier care outside of hospitals by means of mobile coronary care units. Though such schemes had begun in 1966 there was little evidence that they were generally accepted, and in Great Britain only a few were operating, often with difficulty. There had been experiments in training ambulance drivers and firemen to give emergency care and some industrial firms had provided coronary care units in their sick bays.

The general practitioner was somewhat confused about the part he should play and as the doctor of first contact in most cases, he had no generally accepted idea of what to do. A few groups of general practitioners had begun to experiment with their own versions of emergency care and were claiming that they were often able to reach patients more quickly than a coronary ambulance. Some were geared to early transfer to coronary care units while others were prepared to keep patients at home or in cottage hospitals.

Abroad, notably in North America, coronary care was seen mainly in hospital terms. In Britain there was evidence that many patients were being treated at home, with little fuss and apparent success in most cases. There seemed a need to gather together those who were experimenting in community care, in one form or another, to learn what each was doing and to provide some guide lines for the primary physician, as the general practitioner is now called, perhaps appropriately, in this medical emergency.

Doctors on Teesside (now Cleveland County) had been discussing these problems for some time and they assembled a National Workshop in March 1976. Its aims were to receive evidence from those active in the field of community coronary care and to formulate guide lines for primary physicians working in different areas, for example, country districts or large towns. A good measure of agreement was reached

11

between those working in coronary care units, with mobile care units, and in general practice, and it seemed important to make their findings and recommendations more widely available. This book is based on the workshop, though additional material has been added to complete the community approach to the treatment of coronary thrombosis from the general practitioner's point of view.

Inevitably, several authors have discussed the same references and made similar points about care. To avoid repetition I have permitted this only where it was essential to complete the understanding of a particular chapter or where it gave a different slant or interpretation.

PART ONE COMMUNITY CARE

1 THE MEANING OF COMMUNITY CARE

Dr Aubrey Colling

Introduction

Over the last forty years various forms of treatment for patients who
have had an acute myocardial infarction (AMI) have come and gone, or
been modified as the result of further research. These methods of treatment all possessed a reasonable theoretical basis and had strong
advocates with plausible, but often poor, support from facts and
figures. For example, a low calorie diet was advocated by Master et al.[1]
who claimed to have halved the fatality in 243 patients treated in
Mount Sinai Hospital, New York. These authors, together with many
others, were also devoted to prolonged bed rest for their cases which
careful evaluation has now shown to be of no value. [2,3,4] Similarly, the
use of anticoagulant therapy was first reported in 1948[5] and became
the cornerstone of treatment for two decades until the Medical Research
Council Working Party Report[6] failed to demonstrate any reduction in
fatality in a randomised trial. A régime of potassium, glucose and insulin
was found to be helpful by Mittra[7] but a controlled trial by Pentecost[8]
failed to confirm his results. Streptokinase[9,10,26] and aspirin[11,12] are
currently under surveillance in a similar way.

Such a historical to and fro is mentioned to illustrate our present
dilemma. We have now relying increasingly on yet another form of
treatment, the coronary care unit. These units are expensive, both
financially and in medical manpower, yet they have been widely
adopted on unsatisfactory evidence of their value. Hofvendahl[13], for
example, claims that it costs twice as much to care for a patient in a
coronary care unit than on an ordinary ward. More detailed discussion
of these points follows in the next chapter. It is of interest that most of
those who have written about coronary care in the community have been
hospital physicians, usually cardiologists, most of whom have seen the
problem in terms of hospital treatment. Oliver [14] calculated the number
of coronary care beds needed for the City of Edinburgh. More recently
Bloom and Peterson[15,16] have made similar estimations for Massachu-
setts, and call for the surrender of patients by family doctors to the
cardiologists in the coronary care units. An extension of this approach
has been the mobile coronary care unit, as in Belfast, and elsewhere, in
an attempt to reach patients sooner after an attack and to transfer them

to hospital.

As Acheson notes (Chapter 2), there has been only one controlled (but not randomised) comparison of cases treated in coronary care units and in ordinary hospital wards, and no wholly satisfactory experiment comparing home and coronary care unit treated cases. What evidence there is on home care has received more critical appraisal than that for hospital care, and is discussed in detail in the following two chapters.

Hospital Orientation

As an example of where such hospital-orientated thinking leads, the choice of place for treatment of patients in the Teesside survey can be cited.[7] It has been tacitly understood that young men should be preferentially admitted to coronary care units after attacks of AMI. This is confirmed in the admission figures when assessed on a community basis. It can be seen (Figure 1) that the coronary care unit receives a much younger population than either the ordinary hospital wards or

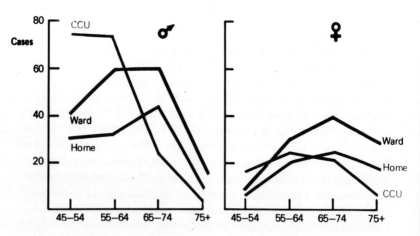

Figure 1 Effect of age on place of treatment (Teesside Coronary Survey). Coronary care units treated more of the younger patients despite their having a lower fatality than older people.

home, a group which is known to have a low fatality rate. Such a policy is illogical unless the community has decided to put all its effort into saving those of special economic value, or it can be shown that this group benefits from intensive care.

The Teesside Coronary Survey, however, failed to demonstrate any benefit from this policy. Figure 2 shows that the fatality of patients is more closely related to age than to where the patient is treated.

**Effect of Age and Place of Admission on Fatality
(Definite Myocardial Infarction)**

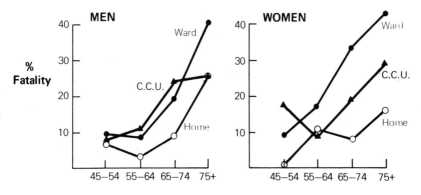

Figure 2 Effect of age on place of treatment and fatality (Teesside Coronary Survey). Although younger patients tended to be admitted to coronary care units this practice did not result in a lower fatality rate by comparison with those treated in ordinary wards or at home.

Mobile Coronary Care Unit (MCCU)

Extending coronary care into the pre-hospital phase, which began in Belfast in 1966, greatly increased our understanding of the autonomic onslaught in the early hours after an infarction and is described by Dr Adgey in Chapter 7. The almost complete elimination of death in transit to hospital and the correction of dysrhythmias in the home are impressive. The fact that patients who have suffered a clinically mild infarction are just as likely to have a cardiac arrest as those who have had a severe attack is a warning to the public and general practitioners not to be unduly sanguine.[18] It raises problems when we try to define the form that primary care should take in different communities (Chapter 11). Cases which on clinical grounds appear to be mild and eligible for home care could die unexpectedly. The various risks must be taken into consideration and are discussed later.

The convincing results reported from some MCCUs should not deter observers from insisting that they should be assessed on a community basis. There are words of caution from the Belfast workers[7] who have shown that a third of patients being transferred to hospital had a heart rate inappropriately rapid which was likely to affect adversely the extent of the infarct. They found frequent ventricular dysrhythmias related to this increased heart rate during the transport of patients.

An interesting evaluation of a cardiac ambulance was made by Hampton[7] in Nottingham who demonstrated the value of assessment on a community basis. The fatality rate of those transferred to hospital by coronary ambulance was 40 per cent, compared to 51 per cent in patients transferred by ordinary ambulance when the coronary ambulance was not available; a difference which seemed to indicate that patients transported by the special vehicle fared better than those brought in by the routine ambulance. But the fatality among patients brought in by the ordinary ambulance when the cardiac vehicle was available but not used was 68 per cent. Under these circumstances the combined fatality rate for all patients brought to hospital by both coronary and ordinary abulance was 51 per cent, a rate identical to that of patients brought in by the routine service when the cardiac vehicle was not available. The explanation appeared to be that when the cardiac vehicle was available there was an unintentional selection of relatively low risk patients for it. Further investigation showed that the difference in fatality rates was due more to patient selection than ambulance crew performance.

Community Surveys

Clearly, great care must be taken when interpreting results. The provision of an MCCU, or other new service, is likely to alter the habits of doctors in the area who will refer a different group of patients in a new way. There is evidence from Belfast, Edinburgh and elsewhere that patients are transferred much earlier and as we have seen in Nottingham, there is a subtle selection of patients for this kind of care. If the Teesside findings are similar to those found elsewhere, which seems likely, then when special facilities are provided they may be given selectively to young people, who are known to have a relatively good outlook.

To overcome these difficulties, it will be increasingly important to assess results on a community basis, incorporating data from hospitals, general practitioners and industry. This has been attempted in four areas in Great Britain, Oxford,[21] Edinburgh,[22] London[23] and Teesside (now Cleveland)[17] with varying degrees of success (Table 1).

The higher incidence in Northern and Scottish communities is already well known and as Taylor pointed out,[24] contrary to what is commonly believed, coronary thrombosis is not a disease of affluence. Rather it occurs in people moving from a state of poverty towards relative affluence. He compared the distribution of affluence in Great Britain in both infant fatality and deaths from ischaemic heart disease. The most affluent areas of Britain were in the South-east of England, where the lowest infant fatality rate was found and also the lowest number of deaths from ischaemic heart disease. Infant fatality is a useful health index and where it is high, as in northern industrial areas and in Scotland, so too are deaths from ischaemic heart disease.

About 5 per cent of attacks begin at work, and though the numbers are small they are probably recognised early and at a time when patients may be unstable and unfit to move. Any concept of community care must include this group of patients and medical departments in industry can be of considerable help, as described by Dr Mayes in Chapter 9.

When we turn to treatment we can see clearly the importance of the community approach. We have seen that special forms of care attract a restricted group of patients and it becomes impossible to interpret their results, unless they can be related to the whole community. The results of the Teesside survey, reported in Chapter 3, came as a surprise. More cases were founded to be treated at home than expected and they differed from those who were sent to hospital in a way not measurable by the usual parameters. In addition, the low fatality found in home-treated cases could not be explained by the fact that less severely ill patients were being cared for at home. Such results were difficult to accept and even harder to interpret, yet demonstrated the value of the epidemiological approach.

Could these results be improved? Those who advocate various forms of care must ensure that there is a solid base of information with which to compare it and anyone suggesting a new treatment must give convincing proof of benefit: this should usually be assessed on a broad community basis. It will no longer be accepted to give figures from

Table 1: Incidence and Fatality in Coronary Thrombosis: Four British Community Studies

	Male								Female								28 Day Fatality		
	20–39	40–49	50–59	60–69	70–79	80–89	90+	40–69	20–39	40–49	50–59	60–69	70–79	80–89	90+	40–69	Male	Female	Male & Female
Oxford pop. 375,000	0.4	2.7	5.7	13.0				6—7	0	0.2	1.0	3.9							59% (20—69)
Edinburgh pop. 500,000	0.59	6.55	16.51	25.54				15	0.14	1.41	4.29	10.0					32.6	33.0	32.7% (20—69)
Tower Hamlets London pop. 82,200 (Aged 25–64)		1.6 (25—44)	10.0 (45—64)					10 (45—64)		0.2 (25—64)		2.7 (25—64)					2.7 (45—64)		40% (—69)
Teesside pop. 396,000	1.6 (30—39)	5.1	14.1	26.0	33.9	40.4	30.8	13.4	0.2 (30—39)	1.6	5.6	10.7	20.2	28.2	60.2	5.5	49.3	51.4	50.5% (All ages)

hospital cases only, or from MCCUs, without placing them in a more general context. All physicians can quote success stories of the resuscitation of individual patients in coronary care units. Against this must be balanced the possible harm of interference in any way with the natural history of the condition and simple symptomatic treatment, such as the relief of pain. There is good evidence that some interference is helpful, but these measures are not without risk and it will be essential in the future to show that they can be applied on a community basis to improve fatality.

Some Problems of Community Care

Because of geographical and other local considerations, no universal plan can be suggested for the care of patients after myocardial infarction. Some general practitioners work at a great distance from the nearest hospital. Most large hospitals now contain coronary care units but they are sometimes poorly staffed and organised, and have been criticised even by those who advocate them. Despite the known high early mortality after myocardial infarction there has been little local or national propaganda to educate the public. The only success has been the reduction in the time of notification of cases following the introduction of a coronary ambulance, as in Belfast and Edinburgh. Coronary ambulances have not been generally accepted, however, partly because of shortage of staff and money, and partly because of the lack of conviction as to their value. While such caution is laudable, it is not matched by any great concern for patients being transferred from home to hospital without adequate monitoring in the first two or three hours after an attack. As the public becomes more aware of the urgency in receiving treatment, so delays will be less, and the general practitioner will see more of the early cases with unstable rhythms and autonomic imbalance. Moving such patients in ordinary ambulances without monitoring and resuscitative facilities would seem to be fraught with danger and we need local initiative to overcome this lack of facilities.

What Is the Possible Saving of Life?

Figure 3 shows the overall picture on Teesside where 50 per cent of patients died within twenty-eight days. The mean time for patients coming under care was three hours, the fatality rate by then being 43 per cent. As things stand at present, therefore, any extra saving of life must come from this 7 per cent of patients who died after coming under care. The nature of the graph (Figure 3) in the first three hours is not accurately known and better community surveys are needed to determine whether extra effort applied in the first few hours would be worth the cost and troubled involved. There is a danger that the groups of doctors who are beginning to provide special care are doing so as a matter of faith and in a way which will prove difficult to evaluate.

TEESSIDE CORONARY SURVEY

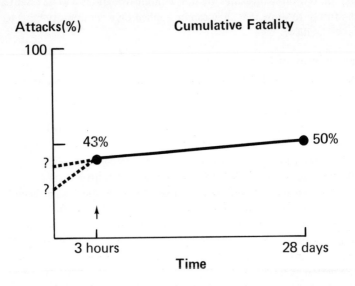

Figure 3 Comulative fatality rate (Teesside Coronary Survey). 50 per cent of patients suffering a myocardial infarction died within twenty-eight days of the attack. After three hours 43 per cent had died, that is by the median time for patients coming under care. Treatment was given therefore to just over half the cases.

Pantridge and his colleagues[25] say that the addition of the MCCU to the coronary care unit in the community is likely to treble the saving of life achieved, but the calculations are highly speculative and based on selected patients.

Whatever the arguments may be on the merits of one form of care against the other, it has become clear that future advances will be in the community and not in hospital. The challenge, therefore is to the general practitioner, to the ambulance services and to those in hospital who will turn out to help. The purpose of this book is to place the problems before the family doctor to see whether he is prepared to rise to the challenge. Does he see himself in the front line of this epidemic?

Notes

1. Master A.M. *et al.*, The Treatment and the Immediate Prognosis of Coronary Artery Thrombosis (267 Attacks)', *American Heart Journal,* 1936, 12, pp.549-62.
2. Medical Division, Glasgow Royal Infirmary, 'Early Mobilisation After Uncomplicated Myocardial Infarction', *Lancet,* 18 August 1973, pp.346-9.
3. Harpur J.E. *et al.,* 'Controlled Trial of Early Mobilisation and Discharge from Hospital in Uncomplicated Myocardial Infarction', *Lancet,* 18 December 1971, pp.1331-4.
4. Lamers H.J. *et al.,* 'Early Mobilisation after Myocardial Infarction: A Controlled Study, *British Medical Journal,* 1973, 1, pp.257-9.
5. Wright I.S., Marple C.D. and Beck D.F., 'Anticoagulant Therapy of Coronary Thrombosis with Myocardial Infarction,' *Journal of the American Medical Association,* 1948, 138, pp.1074-9.
6. Medical Research Council Working Party, 'Assessment of Short-term Anticoagulant Administration After Cardiac Infarction', *British Medical Journal,* 1969, 1, pp.335-42.
7. Mittra B., 'Potassium, Glucose and Insulin in the Treatment of Myocardial Infarction', *Lancet,* 1965, ii, p.607.
8. Pentecost B.L. *et al.,* 'Controlled Trial of Intravenous Glucose, Potassium and Insulin in Acute Myocardial Infarction', *Lancet,* 4 May 1968, pp.946-8.
9. European Working Party, 'Streptokinase in Recent Myocardial Infarction: A Controlled Multicentre Trial', *British Medical Journal,* 1971, 3, pp.325-31.
10. Bett J.H.N. *et al.,* 'Australian Multicentre Trial of Streptokinase in Acute Myocardial Infarction', *Lancet,* 13 January 1973, pp.57-60.
11. Boston Collaborative Drug Surveillance Group, 'Regular Aspirin Intake and Acute Myocardial Infarction', *British Medical Journal,* 1974, 1, pp.440-3.
12. Elwood P.C. *et al.,* 'A Randomised Controlled Trial of Acetyl Salicylic Acid in the Secondary Prevention of Mortality from Myocardial Infarction', *British Medical Journal,* 1974, 1, 436-40.
13. Hofvendahl S., 'Influence of Treatment in a Coronary Care Unit on Prognosis in Myocardial Infarction', *Acta Medica Scandanavica,* Supplement 519.
14. Oliver M.F., Julian D.G. and Donald K.W., 'Problems in Evaluating Coronary Care Units', *The American Journal of Cardiology,* 1967, 20, pp.465-74.
15. Bloom B.S. and Peterson O.L., 'End Results, Cost and Productivity of Coronary Care Units', *New England Journal of Medicine,* 1973, Vol.288, No.2, pp.72-8.
16. Bloom B.S. and Peterson O.L., 'Patient Needs and Medical-Care Planning. The Coronary Care Unit as a Model', *New England Journal of Medicine,* 1974, Vol.290, No.21, pp.1171-7.
17. Colling W.A. *et al.,* 'Teesside Coronary Survey: An Epidemiological Study of Acute Attacks of Myocardial Infarction', *British Medical Journal,* 1976, 2, pp.1169-72.
18. McNee B.T. *et al.,* 'Long-term Prognosis Following Ventricular Fibrillation in Acute Ischaemic Heart Disease', *British Medical Journal,* 1970, 4, pp.204-6.
19. Mulholland H.C. and Pantridge J.F., 'Heart Rate Changes During Movement of Patients with Acute Myocardial Infarction', *Lancet,* 22 June 1974, pp.1244-7.
20. Hampton J.R., 'Importance of Patient Selection in Evaluating a Cardiac Ambulance Service', *British Medical Journal,* 1976, 1, pp.201-3.
21. Kinlen L.J., 'Incidence and Presentation of Myocardial Infarction in an English Community', *British Heart Journal,* 1973, 35, pp.616-22.
22. Armstrong A. *et al.,* 'Natural History of Acute Coronary Heart Attacks. A Community Study', *British Heart Journal,* 1972, 34, pp.67-80.
23. Pedoe H.T. *et al.,* 'Coronary Heart Attacks in East London', *Lancet,*

1 November 1975, p.833.
24. Taylor Lord, 'Poverty, Wealth and Health, or Getting the Dosage Right', *British Medical Journal*, 1975, 4, pp.207-11.
25. Pantridge J.F. *et al., The Acute Coronary Attack*, Pitman, 1975.
26. Aber C.P. *et al.,* 'Streptokinase in Acute Myocardial Infarction: A Controlled Multicentre Study in the United Kingdom', *British Medical Journal*, 1976, 2, pp.1100-4.

2 THE EFFECTIVENESS OF CARE OF ACUTE MYOCARDIAL INFARCTION: A REVIEW FROM THE EPIDEMIOLOGICAL VIEWPOINT

Professor R.M. Acheson

The Problem

The most important single factor which impedes the bringing of effective treatment to those who have suffered an acute myocardial infarction (AMI) is the urgent need for haste, as can be seen in Figure 1. The data on which the figure is based are derived from one of several major community studies which have been undertaken in the United Kingdom, namely the one carried out in Edinburgh.[1]

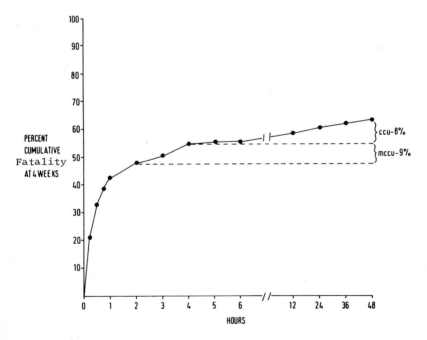

Figure 1 Estimated case fatality rate due to dysrhythmias expressed as a percentage of all deaths occurring in the first four weeks after an acute myocardial infarction. The dotted lines are drawn to indicate that if all cases were admitted to a coronary care unit within 4 hours, the case fatality rate might be reduced by 8 per cent, and that if a mobile coronary care unit could reach all cases within 2 hours of the attack, case fatality rates might be reduced a further 9 per cent.

In the first two hours nearly 50 per cent of those who will die in four weeks have died. This clearly indicates that if something is to be done, it must be done extremely quickly. The biases in the various studies which have sought to examine the effectiveness of medical care, and to which reference will be made, are largely derived from when, on this curve, a patient has an opportunity to avail himself of cardiac resuscitation and such other treatment as he should need. Deaths occurring during the first month divide themselves into three groups. The most important and largest is the group of deaths due to ventricular fibrillation. The size of the group is not known but it is certain that the figure exceeds 35 per cent and may be higher than 70 per cent, and it is these patients for whom something can be done. Some other patients die as a result of shock and hypotension, and the remainder from a variety of such lethal conditions as asystole, cardiac rupture, etc. Thus, the administration of DC shock has made it possible for a significant proportion of people 'dying' soon after an AMI to be brought back from the dead.

Nevertheless, it would now seem that the investment in services we have made in this country in an attempt to make DC shock as widely available as possible may have been made with insufficient evidence. Outstanding questions remain which are never likely to be answered. It is, however, very easy to be wise after the event.

Oliver [2,3] has calculated that if the patient is reached between two and four hours and given the sort of treatment available in coronary care units (CCUs) — which, by and large, at the time he collected the data, meant giving DC shock — the maximum by which the death rate can be reduced is 8 per cent. If the patient can be reached in less than two hours there is a further maximum potential for a 9 per cent reduction in the death rate. Most of this paper is concerned with an attempt to assess what has been done for patients reached between two and four hours; first, however, let us review some of the evidence which amply bears out the belief that the administration of DC shock is effective in the longer as well as the shorter term.

The Outcome of Successfully Resuscitated Ventricular Fibrillation

We conducted a long-term follow-up study at Oxford, through the kindness of Dr Grant Lee and Professor Sleight, of 92 per cent of 330 patients treated for myocardial infarction in the CCU in 1971 to 1972, early in the CCU's existence.[4] Records were complete for 300 of these patients who had suffered a first attack; DC shock was given to 27. Only 60 per cent of the 300 survived for three years, compared with an expected figure of 91 per cent in the general population, a sober reminder that suffering an AMI, with or without defibrillation, is a serious matter. The three-year survival rate of those who received DC shock was 37 per cent.

Information about return to work among men of employable age is shown in Figure 2. It can be seen that 83 per cent of those who did not require shock were working before the attack compared with 91 per cent of those who received it. Seventy-three per cent and 55 per cent respectively returned to work, 55 per cent and 36 per cent to the same job. Although the chances of returning to work after an attack are therefore not so good for those patients who have required shock treatment as for those who have not, it remains impressive. Among other follow-up studies which bear out these findings are those of Cobb,[5] Kushnir[6] and McNamee and his colleagues,[7] which indicate

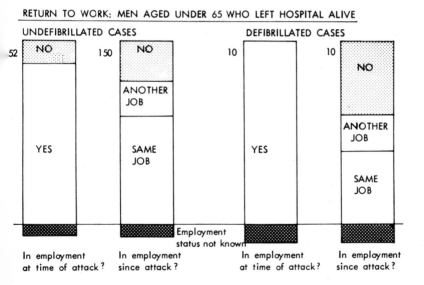

Figure 2 Rates of return to work after an acute myocardial infarction among men aged under sixty-five who left hospital alive. The numbers are few, but it can be seen that although some men who survived ventricular fibrillation returned to their old job, their rates of return to work were not so high as it was among those who did not require defibrillation.

that, granted resuscitation, the nature and magnitude of the infarct may be a more important factor in prognosis than the fact that there was ventricular fibrillation.

There thus can be no doubt about what DC shock offers in terms of long-term survival and as a means of providing people who would otherwise have died with an opportunity of continuing a useful life.

Care between Two and Four Hours; Hospital or CCU?

It can be concluded from the foregoing that it is reasonable to act on an assumption that because the administration of DC shock has the power to bring people back from the dead, the more who can be offered the treatment the better; *post hoc* evidence has shown that their subsequent life has been useful to themselves and to others. Nevertheless, with the notable exception of the study conducted by Mather and his colleagues in the West of England[8,9] to which we shall return, there have been no prospective investigations of the overall implications of concentrating acute coronary care on CCUs and few really satisfactory data are available. For instance, there has never been a randomised trial to determine whether CCUs are more effective at saving lives than other hospital wards and there is now a real question as to whether *on an overall population basis* hospitals can offer better care than the GP who looks after his patient at home. Reasoning backwards from haphazardly collected data has made it incredibly difficult to come to a satisfactory conclusion about such important issues.

It would seem that Hofvendahl[10] has produced the best data available to us comparing general ward with CCU. He worked in a hospital in Stockholm where the CCU was too small to manage every patient requiring care, with the result that cases could only be admitted when beds were available. The other patients went into the general wards. In order to determine whether there were important systematic differences which could influence case fatality rates in the two groups, he compared the patients treated in the CCU with the others in the general wards in terms of age, sex, previous heart diseases, diabetes, pulmonary oedema, left ventricular failure, shock, low blood pressure and the Peel Index. He was unable to find any evidence of bias with respect to any of those factors. Some of Hofvendahl's findings are shown in Table 1 which compares these with other similarly collected data from other countries. It can be seen that in Stockholm 17 per cent of patients in the CCU died in hospital, as opposed to 35 per cent in the general wards. Hofvendahl also found, after three years' follow-up, that age-adjusted cumulative survival rates were about 60 per cent among those treated

Table 1: Observed In-Hospital Case Fatality Rates in Coronary Care Units and General Wards in Several Studies

	Coronary Care Unit		General Ward	
	No. of cases observed	% Died	No. of cases observed	% Died
Edinburgh*	271	14	257	16
Stockholm[10]	132	17	139	35
Tower Hamlets[12]	184	13	211	15
Teesside[11] **	324	14	397	21

* Interpreted by Professor D.G. Julian from the Armstrong *et al.* (1972) study. Julian[13] writes '. . .the figures refer to those cases treated in hospital who were involved in the survey and are accurate', but adds that no attempt was made to randomise patients to the two groups between which there are important differences.
**Death rates are age standardised and include all age groups.

Table 2: Case Fatality Rates from Acute Myocardial Infarction in Home and Hospital According to General Practitioners' Policy for Managing Case[11]

GP's Policy	Actual place of treatment	No. of cases	Case fatality rates	
A. Refer to hospital	Hospital	275	16.7	
	Home	11	18.8	16.8
B. Judged by merits of each case	Hospital	423	17.0	
	Home	359	6.7	12.3

in the CCU, compared with 40 per cent among those treated on the wards. It is important to note that although data relating to case fatality rates in hospital are not strictly comparable with each other, in every instance the case fatality rate is higher in the ward than in the CCU. This is to be expected, but in view of the demands made on resources by CCUs it is a pity that we are unlikely ever to have better information on the matter.

Table 2 presents some data from Teesside[11] which show that the overall case fatality is much lower in those practices (Group B) in which the doctor decides where to treat his patient on the merits of the case than in those (Group A) in which the general policy is to refer all cases to hospital if possible. It is a matter of interest that in the Group B practices the case fatality rate is a little lower than those recorded for CCUs in Table 1. This comparison should be made with caution. The age structures of the Edinburgh, Stockholm and Tower Hamlets populations certainly differed from the Teesside study which considered all the population, even its oldest inhabitants. Another problem is that AMIs, which appeared to be mild, may have been kept at home in the former three communities.

The low case fatality rate in the Group B practices in general, and especially among those kept at home, could therefore be the result of clinical judgement or of bias, but the implication that it may not always be beneficial to be admitted to hospital is supported by the data presented in the following chapter, which indicates that when severity of the attack is taken into account patients still did better at home.

An earlier study on this subject to which I have already alluded has engendered a great deal of controversy. It was a trial conducted by Mather and his colleagues[8,9] which studied how the outcome of home treatment compared with that of hospital treatment. The investigators used random procedures to determine whether a person diagnosed by a general practitioner as suffering an AMI should be cared for in hospital or at home; for obvious reasons, however, a patient could only be admitted to the trial if he and his doctor consented to accept a random decision. There was consent in only about 30 per cent of the cases, the decision in the other 70 per cent being made either by the doctor and/or by the patient in exactly the same way as it had always been made. Thus, if we accept that a controlled trial can only be justifiably considered to be randomised when all or practically all decisions are taken at random, this does not qualify because less than one third of decisions were taken in this way. Nevertheless, in my opinion this trial cannot be dismissed lightly.

The 1976 report showed that in the first week, of the 226 patients randomly allocated to be treated at home eight (4 per cent) died compared with fifteen (7 per cent) of 224 allocated to go to hospital. After 28 days the case fatality rates were 12 per cent and 14 per cent for the home and hospital groups respectively and 20 per cent and 27 per cent after 330 days. These differences are not significant at the 5 per cent level although they approach significance. Thus although there is no evidence of real advantage from being treated at home there is certainly no evidence that being treated there is any worse than being treated in hospital. The proportion of cases of AMI followed by hypotension was, however, smaller in the randomised group than in the rest of the defined population. But a very important feature of the study was that the patients who were not randomised were followed up too. Thus, we have information about the 70 per cent who were not randomised which is comparable to what we have about the others. The 28-day case fatality for patients with hypotension (BP < 100 mg Hg) was 44 per cent if they were randomised to home treatment and 55 per cent if home treatment was selected; corresponding figures for hospital treatment were 47 per cent and 49 per cent respectively. These differences are not statistically significant. As might be expected, low blood pressure carried with it a much worse prognoses than normotension, but with the normotensives the prognoses in the randomised and non-randomised groups was again closely similar. Thus it is difficult to accept that the failure of the authors to demonstrate that any advantage arises from hospital treatment can be attributed to the lack of co-operation obtained from the 70 per cent of the study population which would not accept random allocation of treatment.

Getting the Patient to Hospital

In our Oxford study the need for DC shock was found to be related to the distance from the hospital that the patient lived. Six of the 106 (6 per cent) living in Oxford and 19 of the 175 (11 per cent) who came from the environs required DC shock, and the death rate was also higher among those patients who had to undertake the longer ambulance journey to hospital. Although these differences are large they are not significant. In order to estimate the proportion of people sent to hospital according to distance travelled we used the data from Kinlen's[14,15] study of Oxford — the first of the community studies done in this country.* Among patients aged 35-44 years virtually everyone living in

* In his original work Kinlen used age groupings of 30-39, 40-49 years, etc. For the purpose of our study he kindly recalculated his incidence rates in five-year age groups.

Oxford was referred to hospital but the proportion fell off with increasing age to 29 per cent among those aged 65-69 years. However, the proportion of referrals among those living outside Oxford was much lower in every age group, and ranged from 51 per cent to 16 per cent. If we can take mortality data as an index of incidence, it seems that the incidence of ischaemic heart disease is probably higher in Oxford city than in the environs, but these differences are not sufficient to explain differences in referral patterns. Nor, to judge by census data, would it seem that differences in quality and standards of housing are likely to be responsible. Patients are thus being selected to take the ambulance journey to hospital, which is not surprising, but the reasons for selection are obscure.

We tried to quantify the magnitude of these journeys and used as an index the time taken for an average ambulance journey. Estimates were made by the staff of the Oxford ambulance depot, of average times taken for journeys from the towns and villages where the patients lived to the Radcliffe Infirmary in Oxford. These were originally prepared for Kinlen, but were kindly made available to us. The results are shown in Figure 3 and it can be seen that the case fatality rate is twice as high for people who have to travel a long distance as it is for those who lived in Oxford, this despite the fact that the longer the distance, the greater the time that will have elapsed after the attack and therefore, as Figure 1 shows, the greater will be the chance of survival. There were irregular variations within these extremes which are now shown and which may be due to differences between the criteria by which groups of general practitioners choose patients to go to hospital, to random variation or to other causes. The general trend is clear, however, and it is worth noting that in the three-year follow-up period, survival differences between groups had disappeared. Estimates of the referral rates indicate that these decrease with distance travelled. Thus it seems that in Oxfordshire, journeys to the CCU from rural areas are associated with an increased chance of untoward outcome. It is not clear to what extent this can be attributed to case selection by the general practitioner, to the journey itself or to other factors. One is tempted to argue that the disappearance of a difference in survival is due to the introduction of a premature lethal factor in one group which is absent in the other, whereas the persistence of such a difference would be due to case selection.

Care in Two Hours or Less

Next I would like to turn to some of the work which has been done on

CASE FATALITY RATES BY INDEX OF TIME AND DISTANCE

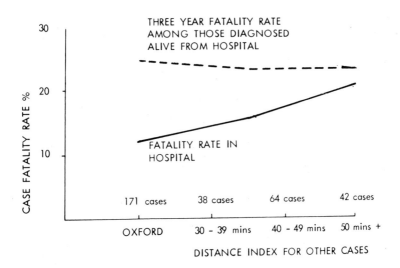

Figure 3 Case fatality rates in hospital, and after three years, according to the estimated duration of the ambulance journey. In each instance observed rates for journeys lasting 30-39 minutes and 40-49 minutes have been averaged.

delivery of care in less than two hours after the onset of an acute myocardial infarction. This has been pioneered among others by Pantridge and his colleagues in Belfast[16] who have concentrated on medically staffed mobile units and in Seattle by Cobb, Baum, Alvarez and Schaffer.[5] Chamberlain has developed a service in Brighton which brings the care to the patient by ambulance manned by a crew which has been specially trained to use electrocardiographic monitors and to treat ventricular fibrillation.[17] The service can be called to the case either by a member of the general public dialling '999', or through a general practitioner.

As long as 1971 the median delay for the ambulance to reach the patient in Brighton was 16 minutes. It took 33 minutes to get the patient to hospital when '999' was dialled, and 121 minutes when a general practitioner was involved, but both have been reduced since then. In the thirteen-month period after Chamberlain started the study, the ambulance was called just over 1,000 times, 667 of which were for cardiac cases. Of these, 65 required the emergency treatment which is appropriate for ventricular fibrillation and 5 of them left hospital alive. Three years later, in 1974, the service answered 1,160 calls in twelve months and the proportions of those requiring DC shock (in one case a thump on the chest restored normal rhythm) as well as the proportions of those being successfully resuscitated by them have increased considerably (see Table 3). When the service started effective resuscitation was provided to 4.6 patients per 1,000 ambulance journeys (about 88 per cent of cases which used the service had heart disease of one sort or another) but with experience, and over a three-year period, this rate has been almost trebled. Now 16.9 per cent of the 160 cases of ventricular fibrillation occuring outside hospital have survived to tell the tale. Thus, Chamberlain and his colleagues have found a method of offering effective help beyond the confines of the CCU to an increasing proportion of those suffering ventricular fibrillation.

Table 3: Two Measures of Efficacy of Brighton Cardiac Ambulance Expressed in Terms of Patients Who Required DC Shock and Left Hospital Alive, Over Two Periods.

In terms of ambulance usage	1971-2 (13 Months)	1974-5 (24 Months)
Successful resuscitation per 1,000 cases carried	4.6	12.0
In terms of medical procedure		
Successful resuscitation — per 100 pulseless cases	7.7	13.0
— per 100 cases of ventricular fibrillation		16.9

Source: White *et al.*, 1973[17]; Briggs *et al.*, 1976[24] and Chamberlain, personal communication.[18]

Conclusion

These studies raise important questions. How, for instance, can an effective service for the care of AMI be developed to take account of population density? Someone living in Oxfordshire may have to spend fifty-five minutes in an ambulance to reach the Radcliffe Infirmary whereas in Brighton and Belfast, where population density is high, travelling time between hospital or ambulance station and patient is short. But a short distance does not necessarily mean a quick journey because another factor is the road system. In some cities there are new limited-access highways which go close to hospitals; in other cities, and in most rural areas, existing road systems are becoming more and more congested, and the sound of the ambulance siren which is needed to get through the traffic could conceivably have an adverse effect on the state of the sick patient carried inside.

What should be the appropriate attitude of the medical profession, and indeed of the trade unions, as to who should man cardiac ambulances? Is it not sensible to have non-medical people staffing them? If so what should their skills, responsibilities and training be?

Even should it be satisfactorily established that it is feasible to care for acute myocardial infarction at home, with or without a mobile unit, cases will still require admission to hospital and the data all suggest that in such instances the specialised care offered by a CCU is beneficial. Between not more than 40 per cent, and in some studies as few as 20 per cent of all cases occur away from home,[4, 12, 19] but some of them much closer to hospital than to their homes and of course there are abundant social reasons why home treatment is undesirable or impossible in other cases even though the attack does occur at home. A CCU, however, is useless unless it is fully manned around the clock by properly trained staff. The costs of this in terms of money and manpower must be balanced against probable case loads and demands upon the hospital for developing in other directions, and Bloom and Peterson[20] have shown that in the Eastern United States there is a strong negative association between case fatality rate and the number of cases treated annually. Here in Britain population density should be taken into account in trying to balance the cost effectiveness equation.

Despite complications the situation is beginning to clarify itself to some extent. Colling[21] has argued that from the clinical standpoint each case of AMI should be treated on its merits, not by rule of thumb, in reaching the answer to the question of 'home or hospital'? I suggest that this is also true in deciding what services a given community should provide for AMI. There is no case, as I see it, for closing all the CCUs in the country – though some people talk along these lines. Nor however can I see that the special committee of the Royal College of Physicians and British Cardiological Society has established a satisfactory case for rapidly increasing the number of CCUs[22]. Districts with hospitals which are without CCUs should think long and carefully before deciding what action is to be taken, and, as I have indicated, should in particular consider such matters as accessibility, population density, probable case loads and the feasibility of various forms of mobile unit which can deliver care at the site of the attack.

We should also ask how many CCUs there should be in any one conurbation and where they should be. We should ask too whether it is worthwhile to try to support them in small, isolated hospitals. Indeed some district general hospitals which have started CCUs may be wise to consider whether they should attempt to retain them. There is ample scope for modification of the Brighton approach with the local cooperation of general practitioners. More *ad hoc* information is needed about the factors which general practitioners actually take into account in deciding how to manage various types of case and in various parts of the country. Hampton[23] and his colleagues in Nottingham have made a start in this direction by surveying opinions from over 200 general practitioners about the way they would approach the management of three hypothetical cases. Our Oxford study raises many interesting questions in this connection, but satisfactory answers can only be obtained by further follow-up articles.

I suspect that I shall look to general practice if I have my coronary at home.

References

1. Armstrong, A. *et al.*, 'Natural History of Acute Coronary Attacks; A Community Study', *British Heart Journal,* 1972, 34, 67-80.
2. Oliver, M.F., Personal communication. 1976.
3. Oliver, M.F., in *Pathogenetic Mechanisms of Angina Pectoris,* ed. Maseri A., New York, 1977. Grune and Stratton.
4. Acheson, R.M. and Sanderson, C.B., 'Some Aspects of the Management and Outcome of Acute Coronary Heart Disease in the Oxford Region', *British Heart Journal,* 1977, 39, 93-8.
5. Cobb, L.A. *et al.*, 'Resuscitation from Out-of-Hospital Ventricular Fibrillation 4 Years Follow-up', *Circulation,* 1975, 51 and 52, Supplement III, 223-8.
6. Kushnir, B. *et al.*, 'Primary Ventricular Fibrillation and Resumption of Work, Sexual Activity and Driving after First Acute Myocardial Infarction', *British Medical Journal,* 1975, 4, 609-11.
7. McNamee, B.T. *et al.*, 'Long-term Prognosis Following Ventricular Fibrillation in Acute Ischaemic Heart Disease', *British Medical Journal,* 1970, 4, 204-6.
8. Mather, H.G. *et al.*, 'Acute Myocardial Infarction: Home and Hospital Treatment', *British Medical Journal,* 1971, 3, 334-8.
9. Mather, H.G. *et al.*, 'Myocardial Infarction: A Comparison between Home and Hospital Care for Patients', *British Medical Journal,* 1976, 1, 925-9.
10. Hofvendahl, S., 'Influence of Treatment in a Coronary Care Unit on Prognosis in Myocardial Infarction', *Acta Medica Scandinavica,* Supplement 519.
11. Donaldson, R.J., Personal communication. 1975.
12. Tunstall Pedoe, H. *et al.*, 'Coronary Heart Attacks in East London', *Lancet,* 1975, 2, 833-8.
13. Julian, D.G., Personal communication. 1976.
14. Kinlen, L.J., 'A Community Study of Acute Myocardial Infarction and Sudden Death', Thesis for D.Phil degree 1969, Bodleian Library, Oxford.
15. Kinlen, L.J., 'Incidence and Presentation of Myocardial Infarction in an

English Community', *British Heart Journal,* 1973, 35, 616-22.

16. Pantridge, J.F. *et al., The Acute Coronary Attack,* London and New York, Pitman, 1975.

17. White, N.M. *et al.,* 'Mobile Coronary Care Provided by Ambulance Personnel', *British Medical Journal,* 1973, 3, 618-22.

18. Chamberlain, D., Personal communication. 1976.

19. Colling, W.A. *et al.,* 'Teesside Coronary Survey: An Epidemiological Study of Acute Attacks of Myocardial Infarction', *British Medical Journal,* 1976, 2, 1169-72.

20. Bloom, B.S. and Peterson, O.L., 'Patient Needs and Medical Care Planning: The Coronary Care Unit as a Model', *New England Journal of Medicine,* 1974, 1171-7.

21. Colling, A., 'Home or Hospital Care after Myocardial Infarction; Is This the Right Question?', *British Medical Journal,* 1974, 1, 559-63.

22. Report of Joint Committee of British Cardiological Society and Royal College of Physicians, 'The Care of the Patient with Coronary Heart Disease', *Journal of the Royal College of Physicians,* 1975, 10, 5.

23. Hampton, J.R., Morris, G.K. and Mason, C., 'Survey of General Practitioners' Attitudes to Management of Patients with Heart Attacks', *British Medical Journal,* 1975, 4, 146-8.

24. Briggs, R. *et al.,* 'The Brighton Resuscitation Ambulance: A Continuing Experiment in Pre-hospital Care by Ambulance Staff', *British Medical Journal,* 1976, 2, 1161.

3 A COMPARISON OF HOME AND HOSPITAL CARE: THE TEESSIDE CORONARY SURVEY

Dr Aubrey Colling and Dr Alexander Dellipiani

Background to Survey

In 1970 a local charity offered a mobile coronary care vehicle to a group of hospital physicians working in a Teesside hospital. The doctors examined the published evidence on the potential benefits of mobile units and were uncertain of their value. Community surveys in Edinburgh[1] and Oxford[2] had shown a great difference in incidence of myocardial infarction but they were deficient in information about old people. Other reports, such as those from Belfast,[3] Bristol[4] and Doncaster, [5] although valuable, were of limited help when considering a community service. A survey in East London[6] was age restricted and had few cases treated at home. Before establishing a service the doctors decided to gather information locally to discover what was already happening to patients after attacks of myocardial infarction. To obtain useful figures it was necessary to study the problem over a period of a year.

Planning took a further two years and the project was financed by the Newcastle Regional Hospital Board. Subsequently the Teesside County Borough Council gave considerable financial support and other help, including computer time. The primary research team consisted of the Medical Officer of Health and his research assistant, two hospital physicians and a general practitioner. They were helped by four full-time nurses with previous experience of intensive care who were given further training in interviewing techniques and epidemiological aspects of the study. A retired industrial scientist acted as coordinator.

Objectives of Survey

The main objectives were to determine,

1. The incidence, mortality and fatality of attacks.
2. The time and place of attacks.
3. The schedule of events leading to patients coming under care.
4. The interval between onset of attacks and death.
5. The frequency and relevance of premonitory symptoms.
6. The fatality of patients treated at home and in hospital.

Data were collected on every suspected case of myocardial infarction reported during the year April 1972-April 1973. The population of Teesside was 396, 000 and was served by 150 general practitioners and 10 consultant physicians working in 14 hospitals, two of which had coronary care units. Cooperation was gained from all family doctors, consultant physicians, emergency medical services, industrial medical officers and nurses attached to family doctors. A simple notification procedure was established which depended on an exclusive telephone with a 24-hour answering service.

Exhaustive efforts were made to ensure that every suspected attack of myocardial infarction was notified. With the cooperation of the registrar of deaths and the coroner all relevant records were made available, as were the records of the emergency medical service and the ambulance service. Each family doctor had a district nurse attached to him responsible to the Medical Officer of Health and she was asked to ensure that all cases of which she was aware were notified. There was considerable local interest in the survey and doctors were encouraged to participate by the ECG reporting service provided throughout the whole study period. They understood that no attempt was being made to interfere with their clinical management and that the information gathered was intended for future planning.

Information was obtained from the patient whenever possible. A survey nurse visited the patient soon after notification and collected personal details of job, age, past history, premonitory symptoms, smoking habits and the timing of events in a standard way. She recorded the pulse and blood pressure, the presence of pallor, cold skin, sweating, confusion, restlessness, dyspnoea and cyanosis. She recorded an electrocardiograph and took blood for serum enzyme estimation. She made a second visit within seventy-two hours, recorded a further electrocardiograph and took blood samples, and sought evidence of oedema, deep venous thrombosis and haemoptysis. If the diagnosis was not firmly established from the results of data collected on the first two visits, a further visit was made on the twenty-eighth day when a third electrocardiograph was recorded. For patients treated in hospital most of this information was abstracted from the patient's record and copies of the cardiographs were obtained. Where patients died suddenly or before the arrival of a survey nurse, the information was obtained from witnesses or from relatives. This particular part of the survey was very time consuming, sometimes embarrassing and after six months was abandoned since it was considered that sufficient information had been collected.

Assessment of Patients

The three clinicians in the research team assessed the information and placed each case in a diagnostic category. The diagnostic categories used and the criteria for ECG changes were based on recommendations of the World Health Organisation[7] and are shown in Table 1.

Table 1: Classification of Myocardial Infarction

		No.	Deaths
Definite MI	A. Evolving injury current on ECG or a typical history with raised enzyme levels plus Q waves, ST changes, T wave changes or bundle branch block.	751	115
	B. Post-mortem evidence of MI or occlusion.	366	366
POSSIBLE MI	A. A typical history of prolonged chest pain associated with a non-diagnostic ECG. The serum enzyme levels might be normal or raised.	333	10
	B. Deaths certified as due to MI	488	488
Not MI	An atypical history with a non-diagnostic ECG and normal serum enzymes. In other cases an alternative diagnosis became obvious after notification or the data were insufficient to permit classification.	833	0

Incidence of Acute Myocardial Infarction

There were 2,771 referrals during the course of the survey year. Of these, 833 were not cases of myocardial infarction. Many of them were false alarms and others had a history which was not typical of a myocardial infarction nor did they have ECG and enzyme evidence to support such a diagnosis (Table 2). The incidence of attacks of myocardial infarction in different age groups is shown in Table 3 and Figure 1 and is seen to be much higher in men than women in most age groups. Under the age of sixty there appears to be a ten-year lag between men and women, increasing to fifteen years over the age of sixty. Though the numbers are small, in the very old it would appear that the incidence in men and women is very similar. Previous

Table 2: Incidence of Attacks of Acute Myocardial Infarction

Final Diagnosis	No.	Annual Incidence Rate (per/1000 population)
Definite MI	1117	2.82
Possible MI	821	2.07
Total Cases	1938	4.89
Not Myocardial Infarction	833	
Total Notifications	2771	

Table 3: Incidence of Attacks of Myocardial Infarction in the Male and Female Population (Definite and Possible MI)

Age (years)	Males			Females		
	Population	Total Cases	Incidence per 1000	Population	Total Cases	Incidence per 1000
-29	100,085	3	0.03	96,775	—	—
30-34	11,785	10	0.8	11,580	1	0.1
35-39	11,720	29	2.5	11,675	4	0.3
40-44	12,845	45	3.5	12,310	9	0.7
45-49	13,105	88	6.7	13,020	32	2.5
50-54	11,315	149	13.2	11,000	44	4.0
55-59	10,060	153	15.2	10,395	77	7.4
60-64	8,835	199	22.5	9,785	83	8.5
65-69	6,975	212	30.4	8,550	114	13.3
70-74	4,420	134	30.3	6,890	130	18.9
75-79	2,420	98	40.5	4,660	104	22.3
80-84	1,190	48	40.3	2,735	70	25.6
85-89	445	18	40.4	1,160	40	34.5
90-94	110	3	27.3	315	20	63.5
95+	20	1	50.0	50	2	40.0
Overall	195,330	*1190	6.1	200,900	*730	3.6

* The data on age and sex were incomplete in a further eighteen cases.

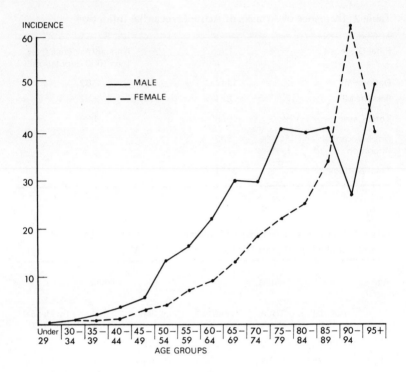

Figure 1 Incidence of attacks of Myocardial Infarction/1000 Population at Risk

community surveys had excluded people over the age of seventy, who were found in this survey to constitute 35 per cent of the total cases.

Place of Treatment

The flow chart (Figure 2) shows what happened to the 1,938 cases of myocardial infarction. 829 patients were untreated and died very quickly (42.8%). Of the remainder approximately the same number of patients were treated at home, on ordinary hospital wards and in coronary care units (Figure 3). No special enquiry was made to determine why doctors chose to keep some patients at home and to send others to hospital. The decision was often made on social grounds where people lived on their own. More single than married people were admitted to hospital. The place of treatment was not influenced by where the attack occurred except for attacks which began in hospital; whether an infarction occurred in the street or at work patients were evenly distributed between the three places of treatment. In other

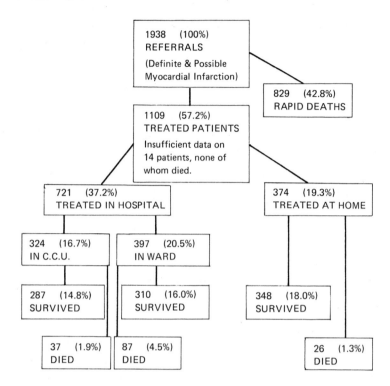

Figure 2 Flow chart showing what happens to the 1,938 patients

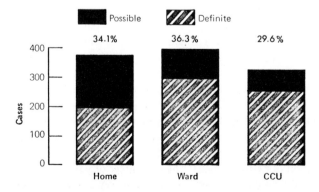

Figure 3 Place of Treatment (1,095 cases)

Table 4: Location of Onset of Attack and Place of Treatment*

Location of onset	Home treated	%	Hospital treated	%	Total	%
Home	289	(34.9)	539	(65.1)	828	(78.1)
Street	30	(37.0)	51	(63.0)	81	(7.6)
Work	23	(32.4)	48	(67.6)	71	(6.7)
Hospital	7	(16.7)	35	(83.3)	42	(4.0)
Other	13	(34.2)	25	(65.8)	38	(3.6)
Total	362	(34.2)	698	(65.8)	1060	(100)

*Total information available for 1060 cases (96 per cent).

words if the attack occurred at work or in the street patients were very often taken home rather than to hospital (Table 4).

Premonitory Symptoms

Though myocardial infarction was first fully described by Obratzow and Straschesko in 1910[8] and by Herrick in 1912[9] it was not until the 1940s that anything was published on prodromal symptoms.[10] There has been increasing interest in what has become known as the 'pre-infarction syndrome', an ill-defined group of symptoms such as shortness of breath, lack of energy, tiredness, indigestion and chest discomfort. Some patients have new or worsening angina and a report from Edinburgh[11] has shown that only about one in six of these patients develop a myocardial infarction. More recently, a prospective study has been made in Rotterdam in a population of more than 20,000 adults.[12] It was found that in an average practice of 3,000 patients some 117 patients per year consulted a general practitioner for 'recent or recently worsened warning symptoms of a coronary event'.

These facts were generally recognised but this study presented a further opportunity to assess their relevance on a community basis. Most patients (76 per cent) had at least one premonitory symptom within ninety days of their infarction and more than one third had consulted their general practitioner in the month before the attack. Twenty per cent of patients experienced either new angina or exacerbation of existing angina. The percentage of patients who experienced premonitory symptoms in the survey as a whole is shown in Table 5.

Table 5: Proportion of Patients Experiencing Premonitory Symptoms
(Definite and Possible Cases)*

	No. (%) of Patients	
Unusual Tiredness	384	(19.8)
Unusual Breathlessness	343	(17.7)
Chest Discomfort	217	(11.2)
Exacerbation of Angina	198	(10.2)
New Angina	198	(10.2)
Heaviness in Arms	171	(8.8)
Unusual Indigestion	140	(7.2)
Palpitations	83	(4.3)

* Within ninety days of attack

Excluding angina, the remainder of these symptoms are common
complaints. Their frequency in the general population was assessed
by taking a sample of sixty-nine cases of definite myocardial infarction
under the age of seventy and comparing them to a similar number of
people taken from the list of a typical general practice matched for age
and sex but excluding those who had a history of myocardial infarction
or angina. Premonitory symptoms were found to be more frequent in
the cases than in the controls (Table 6). It will, however, be recalled
that a number of patients were notified to the survey as cases of
myocardial infarction in whom the diagnosis was subsequently excluded.
The incidence of premonitory symptoms in this group was found to be
even higher than the cases and controls. The reasons for this are not
fully understood but the findings demonstrate the limitations of
premonitory symptoms as diagnostic pointers.

The time relationship of these premonitory symptoms to the onset
of the attack in the three groups is shown in Figures 4, 5 and 6. They
demonstrate a very different pattern between the cases and controls.
However, there was very little difference between cases and those who
turned out not to have had a myocardial infarction ('Not MI'). It could
be argued that the 'Not MI' group had a similar pattern to cases
because they were in a pre-infarction phase, but this was not
substantiated by these patients becoming cases during the course of
this survey. The reason for this similarity has not been explained.

Table 6: Numbers of Patients and Controls Experiencing Certain
General Symptoms*

	Controls N = 69	Patients with Infarction N = 69	Patients without Infarction N = 69
Unusual Tiredness	5	16	18
Unusual Breathlessness	3	11	17
Unusual Indigestion	2	6	13
Chest Discomfort	2	10	9
Heaviness in Arms	1	5	5
Palpitations	1	2	6
Total No. of Patients	8 (11.6%)	30 (43.5%)	41 (56.0%)
Consulted General Practitioner within 90 days	20 (28.9%)	13 (18.8%)	29 (42.0%)

*Within previous ninety days.

Delay Factors

Delay factors have been reported from various surveys (Edinburgh,[1]
Belfast,[3] Doncaster,[5] Barnsley,[13] Oxford[2] and East London[6]) and
are clearly very important both in understanding fatality rates and in
planning a coronary care service. The results of three of these surveys
are shown in Figure 7. They are not intended to be compared
critically since they were widely separated in time and methodology.
The figures from Edinburgh were described before their mobile
coronary ambulance was operating. The Doncaster figures were taken
from selected practices committed to sending their patients to a
coronary care unit. The delays described in the Teesside survey are
restricted to those patients who were notified within twelve hours
of the incident since it would be misleading to include patients who
came under medical care some days after an infarction.

The delays shown in Table 7 include both home- and hospital-treated
cases and analysis showed a considerable difference between them. Just
over one third of patients were kept at home. The sequence of events
was much longer in these cases (Figure 8). The general practitioner was
called to these patients later and, having been called, he took twice as
long to get there when compared to cases he sent to hospital. The result

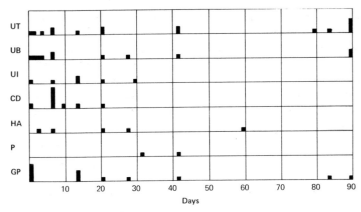

Figure 4 Premonitory Symptoms — Cases

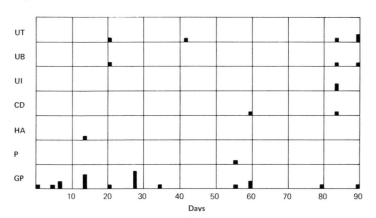

Figure 5 Premonitory Symptoms — Controls

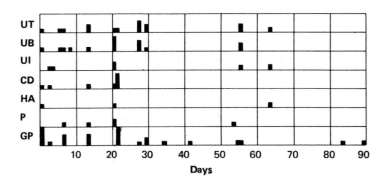

Figure 6 Premonitory Symptoms — Not MI

Table 7: Median Time Delay Periods for Definite and Possible Cases

Time Periods	Definite Cases	Possible Cases	Definite and Possible Cases
Onset – Call GP	1 hour 2 mins.	1 hour 18 mins.	1 hour 11 mins.
Call GP – Arr. GP	29 mins.	46 mins.	30 mins.
Arr. GP – Call Amb.	44 mins.	33 mins.	44 mins.
Call Amb. – Arr. Amb.	13 mins.	13 mins.	13 mins.
Arr. Amb. – Arr. Hpl.	23 mins.	22 mins.	22 mins.
Onset – Arr. Hpl.	2 hours 51 mins.	3 hours 12 mins.	3 hours 0 mins.

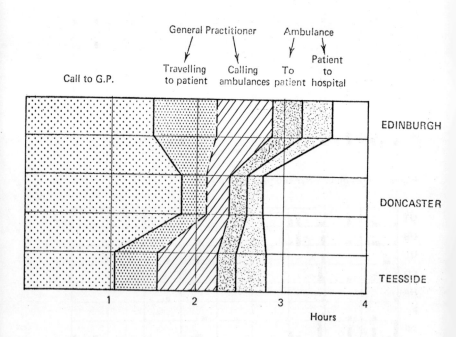

Figure 7 Teesside Coronary Survey. Delay Factors.

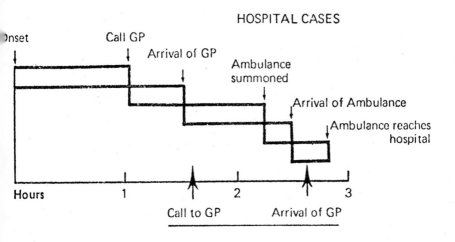

Figure 8 Teesside Coronary Survey. Delay Factors (Median Times)

was that home cases came under the care of their general practitioners
and hospital cases came under hospital care after the same time interval,
that is about three hours. The delay of the ambulance reaching the
patient and transferring the patient to hospital was very short compared
to other delays. When the 'GP delay' is looked at more closely
(Figure 9) it will be seen that without any publicity in the community
the general practitioner was already being called to 50 per cent of cases
within an hour of the onset of attack.

In some cases, of course, the delay was much longer since patients
often called their doctor late without any indication of urgency. The
general practitioner reached more than half the cases in just under two
hours from the onset. What is more important, he arrived within an

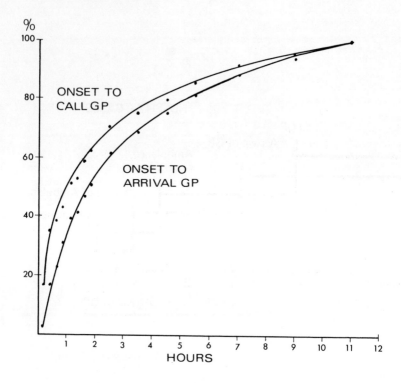

Figure 9 Delay Factors (Cumulative Percentages)

hour of the onset in about a third of patients, at a time of considerable autonomic instability (as described by Dr Adgey in Chapter 7) when special care could possibly lower fatality.

It is difficult to explain the curious difference in the speed of notification in those cases which the general practitioner subsequently sent to hospital, and those he kept at home. In the hospital cases, the general practitioner was, on average, called half an hour earlier and reached the patient twice as quickly. It is possible that this difference may relate to severity in some way, as discussed later. It has been suggested by Professor Julian in Chapter 6 that the mode of onset — sudden or gradual — determines whether a patient will be admitted to hospital or not but this survey showed no significant difference between the two groups (Table 8). Nor was it explained by whether the main symptom was pain, syncope, dyspnoea or dysrhythmia. Possibly it may reflect a patient's pain threshold or be a measure of his or his family's anxiety, though a small enquiry into the anxiety of patients

Table 8: Place of Treatment and Mode of Onset

Onset (%)	Home Treated (%)		Hospital Treated (%)	
Sudden (79.9)	191	(33.8)	571	(66.2)
Gradual (20.1)	80	(36.9)	137	(63.1)

Total information available for 1,079 cases (97.3 per cent).

Table 9: Mortality and Fatality Rates of Myocardial Infarction in Male and Female Population (Definite and Possible MI).

Age Groups	Deaths		Mortality (per 1000)		Fatality (%)	
	Male	Female	Male	Female	Male	Female
-29	—	—	—	—	—	—
30-34	2	—	0.2	—	20.0	—
35-39	6	2	0.5	0.2	20.7	—
40-44	14	2	1.1	0.2	31.1	22.2
45-49	24	12	1.8	1.0	27.3	37.5
50-54	66	15	5.8	1.4	44.3	34.1
55-59	65	20	6.5	1.9	42.5	26.0
60-64	81	32	9.2	3.3	40.7	38.6
65-69	115	45	16.5	5.3	54.3	39.5
70-74	89	83	20.1	12.0	56.4	63.9
75-79	65	68	26.9	14.6	66.3	65.4
80-84	41	50	34.5	17.9	85.4	70.0
85-89	16	33	36.0	28.4	88.9	82.5
90-94	2	13	*	41.3	*	65.0
95+	1	2	*	*	*	*
Missing	5	10				
Overall	592	387	3.0	1.9	49.3	51.4

*Numbers too small to derive reliable rates.

treated at home and in hospital[14] showed no difference on formal testing.

Fatality

The mortality and fatality rates were based on deaths which occurred within twenty-eight days of the onset of the attack. The overall mortality rate (deaths within twenty-eight days per 1,000 population) was 2.5. The overall fatality rate (deaths within twenty-eight days per 100 attacks) was 50.5. A detailed distribution by age and sex is shown in Table 9.

The total number of deaths in men and women of different age groups is shown in Figure 10. When expressed in terms of the percentage of those dying in each group (Figure 11), fatality is seen to increase with age, women having a generally more favourable outcome than men.

Interval between Onset of Attack and Death

Many patients died soon after the attack and as these deaths were frequently unwitnessed it was difficult to obtain information about them. Where deaths had been witnessed evidence of interval from onset to death was obtained in 78 per cent of patients, increasing to 94 per cent in the 'definite' category. In witnessed deaths more than 70 per cent died within three hours of onset, the median time for patients coming under care (Figure 12).

Severity of Cases

The crude fatality rates (Table 10) appeared to favour home care. Ward cases seemed to fare worst of all. A simple explanation for these different fatality rates might have been that there was a difference in the severity of the groups of cases treated. It was essential, therefore, to try and measure the severity of the attack in these patients. The size of the survey and the fact that many cases were treated at home presented us with difficulties and precluded using an index such as the Norris index[15] which includes certain physical signs and measurements such as radiological oedema. The Peel index[16] has been used widely in epidemiological work and seemed appropriate to our study.

The severity index devised by Peel was modified to incorporate information the nurses had obtained and also to include biochemical data (Table 11). The scores given to each of the factors in the modified index were derived from the original Peel index which does not, however, include serum enzyme levels. Appropriate severity scores for the serum aspartate aminotransferase (SGOT) were derived from

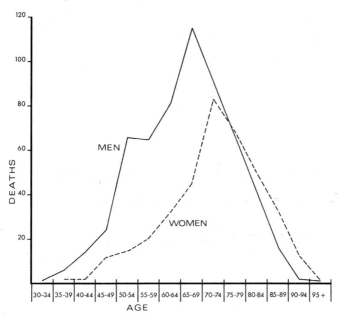

Figure 10 Deaths from Myocardial Infarction (Definite and Possible Cases)

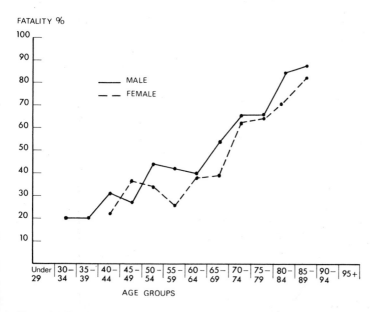

Figure 11 Fatality from Myocardial Infarction (%) (Definite and Possible Cases)

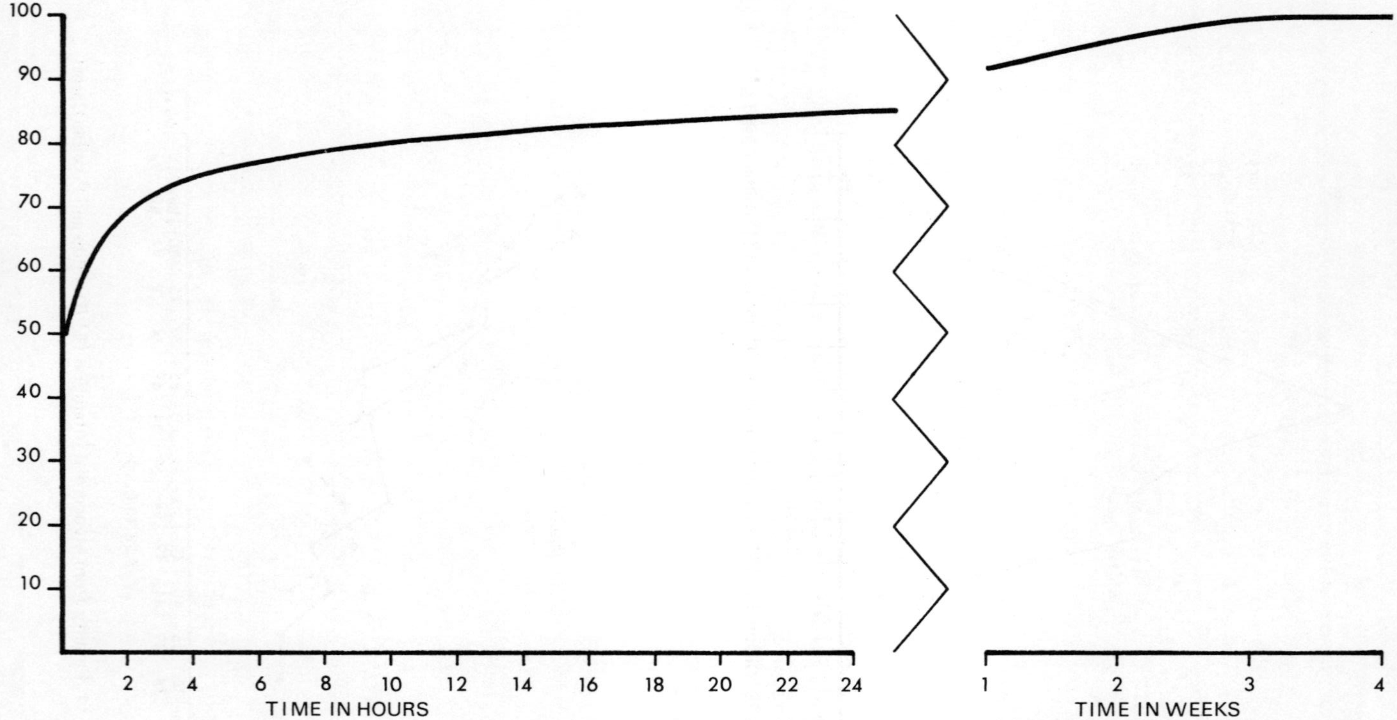

Figure 12 Time of Onset to Death 28 day Cumulative Fatality (Definite and Possible Cases)

Table 10: Crude Fatality Rates (%) in Patients with Definite
Myocardial Infarction*

Place of Treatment	Home	Ward	Coronary Care Unit
Men	8.3	15.8	11.8
Women	9.7	28.6	15.7

*The effect of including 'possible' myocardial infarctions would be to make the difference in the fatality rate between home and hospital care more marked.

literature relating fatality to SGOT levels.[17] ECG criteria for infarction and analyses of rhythm changes were taken from the first ECG and the SGOT level from the initial estimation, either at home or in hospital. The scores obtained were related to fatality defined as death at or within twenty-eight days of the incident.

We confined our study of fatality in relation to severity to those cases who were confirmed as having had a 'definite' myocardial infarction (a well-defined group) and had survived long enough to receive care and have the diagnostic investigations applied (see 'Definite' group A, Table 1). Only one patient who was kept at home died between the time of notification and arrival of the nurse.

In 737 (98 per cent) of the 'definite' group the place of treatment was known (Table 12). The fatality rates are shown in more detail in Tables 13 and 14. It can be seen that relatively young men were selected for treatment in the coronary care unit, a group that is know to have a comparatively low fatality. It will be seen later that this did not appear to benefit these patients.

The Peel Index

The modified Peel index was applied to these cases and the banded scores were plotted against fatality rates (Figure 13). The regression line (p < 0.01), indicated that severity, as measured by the modified Peel index, was related to fatality. The distribution of the modified Peel scores by the three places of treatment is illustrated in Figure 14. The difference in the percentage of patients in each score group treated at home, in the ward and in the coronary care unit did not reach statistical significance.

Table 11:   Modified Peel Index

		Severity Score
Age and Sex		
Male	Female	
< 55 years		0
55-59 years		1
60-64 years	< 65 years	2
> 65 years	> 65 years	3
Past History		
Previous MI		6
Other Cardiovascular Disease or Exertional Dyspnoea		3
Angina only		1
No Cardiovascular Disease		0
Shock		
B.P. > 100 mm Hg		0
B.P. < 100 mm Hg		4
B.P. < 100 mm Hg with cold extremities		7
Failure		
Not Breathless		0
Breathless		4
ECG		
Normal ECG		0
Normal ORS, ST & T wave changes		1
QR		3
QS or BBB		4
Rhythm		
Sinus		0
One or more of:		
Arterial Fibrillation or Flutter; Paroxysmal Atrial Tachycardia; Sinus Tachycardia (>110/min); Frequent Ectopics; Nodal Rhythm or Block		4
SGOT		
< 12 units (Normal)		0
12-60 units		1
> 60 units		4

Table 12:   Place of Treatment for 'Definite' Myocardial Infarctions

Place of Treatment	Home	Ward	Coronary Care Unit	Total
Men	121	184	178	483
Women	72	112	70	254
Total	193	296	248	737

Table 13:   Age — Distribution and Fatality in Home, Ward and CCU (Definite Cases): Males

	Home			Ward			CCU		
Age (years)	Nos.	Deaths	%	Nos.	Deaths	%	Nos.	Deaths	%
45-54	31	2	6.5	41	4	9.8	75	6	8.0
55-64	33	1	3.0	61	5	8.2	74	8	10.8
65-74	45	4	8.9	62	12	19.4	25	6	24.0
> 75	12	3	25.0	20	8	40.0	4	1	25.0
Standardised Fatality %			7.3			14.1			14.6

Table 14:   Age — Distribution and Fatality in Home, Ward and CCU (Definite Cases): Females

	Home			Ward			CCU		
Age (years)	Nos.	Deaths	%	Nos.	Deaths	%	Nos.	Deaths	%
45-54	6	0	0	11	1	8.9	17	3	17.7
55-64	20	2	10.0	30	5	16.7	24	2	8.3
65-74	26	2	7.7	40	13	32.5	22	4	18.2
> 75	20	3	15.0	31	13	42.0	7	2	28.6
Standardised Fatality %			9.0			26.9			17.6

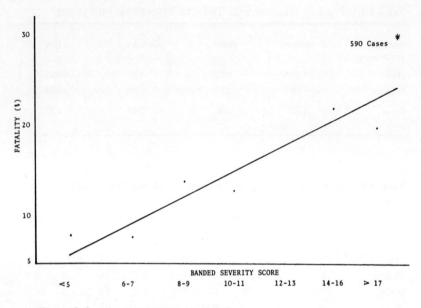

Figure 13 Severity Score Related to Fatality

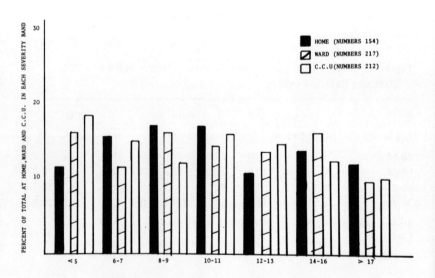

Figure 14 Severity Score Related to Place of Treatment

Individual Severity Factors

The modified Peel index did not reveal any difference in severity
between the patients in the three places of treatment but it is a
relatively insensitive index. In addition, because data was missing in
some cases, modified Peel scores were obtained in only 80 per cent of
patients. It was also suspected that the overall index could mask the
effect of individual factors on fatality. Each factor was therefore
examined independently in relation to fatality. The number of missing
observations for any individual factor were very few indeed — less than
5 per cent in all cases.

Only two factors, a low blood pressure (Table 15) and a past history
of cardiovascular disease (Table 16), were found to be unrelated to
increasing fatality, contrary to the experience of others.[4, 9] All the
other factors in the index — increasing age (Figure 15), heart failure
(Table 17), increasing extent of infarction on ECG (Table 18), rhythm
disturbance (Table 17) and very high SGOT levels (Table 19) — were
associated with statistically higher fatality rates. However, with the
exception of age and very high SGOT levels, these factors were found
to be equally distributed in severity between the home, hospital ward
and coronary care unit cases.

Age

As has been shown (see Table 9), fatality tends to increase with age.
However, it was found that younger patients tended to go into the
coronary care unit. Forty-three per cent of cases in the survey were
over sixty-five years old yet only 19 per cent of them were treated in
the coronary care unit (from Tables 12, 13 and 14). When the crude
fatality rates were standardised for age (see Tables 13 and 14), the
standardised fatality rates in coronary care units were increased and
the better figures for home treated cases remained.

Serum Aspartate Transferase (SGOT — normal level: 12 i.u./litre)

Table 20 shows unequal distribution of SGOT levels in the three places
of treatment, mainly in those patients with very high results (more
than 60 units). Only 24 per cent of patients had such high levels.
Similar standardisation for SGOT had little effect on the crude fatality
rates because of the small numbers of cases with such high levels.

Figure 16 illustrates the increasing fatality with increasing severity
due to age, SGOT and ECG changes and the apparent lack of benefit
from hospital care.

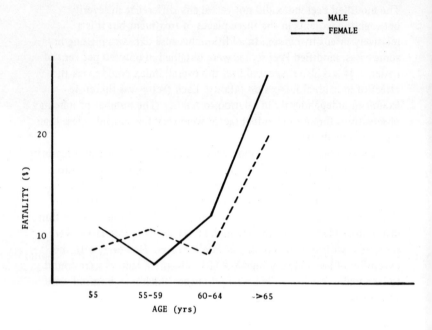

Figure 15 Fatality Related to Age and Sex (Definite Cases)

Table 15:   Fatality Related to Systolic Blood Pressure (Definite Cases)*

			Fatality
>100 mg. Hg	658	(91.3%)	14.3%**
<100 mg. Hg	63	(8.7%)	17.5%**

* Information on 98 per cent of patients.

** Difference not significant.

Table 16:   Fatality Related to Past History ('Definite' Cases)*

Past History	Patients	Patients	Fatality %
Nil		372	15.6
Angina		78	17.9
Other CV Disease		80	15.0
Myocardial Infarction		190	15.8
		720	100

*Information available on 98 per cent of patients.

Table 17:   Fatality Related to Rhythm Disturbance and Heart Failure (Breathlessness) in 'Definite' Cases

	Dysrhythmia		Heart Failure	
	Present	Absent	Present	Absent
Fatality	21.6%	12.4%	20.0%	14.2%

Table 18:   Fatality Related to Extent of Infarction ('Definite' Cases)

ECG Changes	Patients	Fatality %
Normal	157	8.9
Intra-mural	196	11.2
QR	157	21.0
QS: BBB	241	19.1
Total	751*	

*In fourteen cases the place of treatment was unknown.

Table 19:   Fatality Related to SGOT Level ('Definite' Cases)

SGOT i.u./l	Patients	Fatality %
< 12	143	9.1
12-60	399	12.7
> 60	170	23.7
	712	

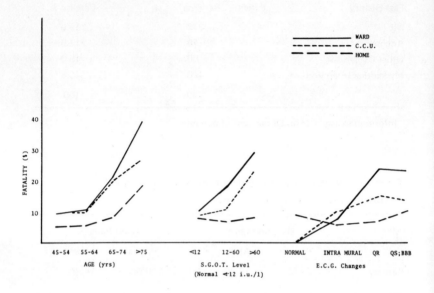

Figure 16 Fatality Related to Age; SGOT and ECG; Ward, CCU and Home.
(Definite cases)

Table 20:   SGOT Distribution and Fatality in Home, Ward and CCU
('Definite' Cases)*

SGOT	Home			Ward			CCU		
(Normal less than 12 i.u./l	No.	Deaths	%	No.	Deaths	%	No.	Deaths	%
< 12	36	3	8.3	48	5	10.5	59	5	9.0
12-60	120	9	7.5	162	30	18.5	117	13	11.1
> 60	26	2	7.7	74	23	31	70	15	21.4
Standardised Fatality %			7.7			19.9			13.1

*Information available on 712 cases (97 per cent).

Comments on Severity

Clearly, the severity of cases in the three places of treatment, apart from the two exceptions mentioned (age and SGOT), were very similar and when the crude fatality rates were standardised for these differences there was a clear advantage for home-treated cases. We have reservations about this type of analysis, particularly the effect of incomplete notification of deaths at home, the different delay factors and the limitations of the objective measurements made. These aspects are discussed later.

Though the ECG findings, analysis of rhythm changes and SGOT estimations were taken from the initial examination for the assessment of severity, a similar analysis was made from the data recorded at a second examination made within seventy-two hours of the onset. The findings did not change the conclusions drawn from the first assessment and allay our concern that a difference in the time since infarction in taking electrocardiographs and blood for enzyme estimation at home and in hospital might influence our results to the advantage of home treated cases.

Social Class

Table 21 compares the social class of patients suffering myocardial infarction to that of the general population on Teesside. Patients in social classes I, II and III had a higher rate of myocardial infarction and those in IV and V a lower rate than expected and these differences were statistically significant. It might have been expected that a patient's social class influenced whether he was treated at home or in hospital, but this was not the case (Table 22).

The Effect of the General Practitioner's Policy on Care

On looking more closely at the way individual doctors managed their patients, it was found that some doctors had a policy of sending almost all their suspected cases of myocardial infarction into hospital whilst others, the majority, adopted a mixed policy, keeping a proportion of cases at home. The age/sex distribution of the patients appeared to be the same in both groups. The doctors' experience, in terms of the year they qualified, and the size of their practices were also similar.

Table 23 shows the fatality rates in these groups of patients. Those doctors who admitted all their cases to hospital had a higher overall fatality rate than those who kept some at home, a difference which, though not strictly statistically significant, shows a trend in favour of

Table 21:   Social Class and the Incidence of Myocardial Infarction

Social Class	No.(%) with Definite Infarction	No.(%) with Possible Infarction	Total (%)	Teesside (at 1971 Census) % Distribution
I	39 (4.7)	25 (4.5)	64 (14.7)	4.1
II	155 (18.8)	84 (15.2)	239 (17.4)	11.5
III	499 (60.5)	319 (57.9)	818 (59.4)	51.1
IV	87 (10.5)	101 (18.3)	188 (13.7)	18.8
V	45 (5.5)	22 (4.0)	67 (4.9)	12.4
Others				2.1
Total	825 (100%)	551 (100%)	1376 (100%)*	100.0

* Information on social class was available for only 71 per cent of patients.

Table 22:   The Place of Treatment and Social Class after Myocardial Infarction

Social Class	No.(%) Treated at Home	No.(%) Treated in Hospital	Total (%)	Teesside (at 1971 Census) % Distribution
I	16 (4.4)	27 (4.2)	43 (4.2)	4.1
II	74 (20.4)	100 (15.5)	174 (17.3)	11.5
III	186 (51.2)	375 (58.2)	561 (55.7)	51.1
IV	75 (20.7)	107 (16.6)	182 (18.1)	18.8
V	12 (3.3)	35 (5.4)	47 (4.7)	12.4
Others				2.1
Total	363 (100%)	644 (100%)	1007 (100%)*	100.0

* Information available on 92 per cent of all treated cases.

Table 23:   Effect of General Practitioner Policy on Fatality Rates

	Total Number of Treated Patients	Overall Fatality Rate
'Hospital Policy' Doctors	286	16.8
'Mixed Policy' Doctors	782	12.3

the group managing their patients at home.

Uptown and Downtown

In the course of various research projects, the Teesside Health Department had compared the health experience of people living in the poorer parts of the town ('Downtown') to those living elsewhere. 'Downtown' made up the old urban core and the remainder was 'Uptown'. The method of defining 'Downtown' depended on three housing characteristics — overcrowding, lack of housing amenities and a higher proportion of private rented accommodation. It had been shown, for example, that the infant mortality in 'Downtown' areas was very high, whilst that in 'Uptown' areas was very low. Taylor[18] has pointed out that areas in Great Britain with a high infant mortality rate also had a high incidence of myocardial infarction. In this survey there did not appear to be any local difference in incidence between the two areas (Table 24) but those in the 'Uptown' area had a more favourable outcome than those living 'Downtown'.

Various factors were studied to see if the difference in fatality between the two zones could be explained — age, sex, civil status, economic status, social class, smoking habits, past history, place of onset of attack and death. As expected there was a significant difference in social class between the two zones and there were more smokers 'Downtown'. Otherwise, there was little difference between the two groups.

Table 24: 'Downtown/Uptown' Incidence, Mortality and Fatality*

	'Uptown'	'Downtown'
Total Cases	1,421	302
Total Deaths	695	166
Total Population	326,494	69,736
Incidence (per 1,000 pop.)	4.4	4.3
Mortality (per 1,000 pop.)	2.1	2.4
Fatality (%)	48.9	55.0

* 'Uptown/Downtown' classification was possible in 89 per cent of cases.

Most of the difference in fatality between 'Uptown' and 'Downtown' areas occurred in the 'possible' group of patients where death had been certified as due to myocardial infarction without post-mortem examination (see 'possible' group B, Table 1). Whether this represented a truly higher fatality 'Downtown' or just a willingness to issue death certificates without post-mortem examination in such circumstances must remain unresolved.

Planning a Community Service

The successful completion of the Teesside survey resulted from the close cooperation between hospital medical staff and those working in the community. Previous surveys had excluded patients over the age of seventy, a serious omission in the context of an aging population, particularly when we were attempting to plan resuscitative facilities for the community. Did the survey influence general practitioner management policy to any significant degree? If it did then the results do not reflect the usual practice at the time. It was our impression, however, that it did not. We might have expected that the survey would orientate coronary management towards the hospital but this did not seem to happen. Indeed, the incidence of home-treated cases (34 per cent) was higher than that of other reports in Britain.[19] Of the rest of the cases approximately one half were treated in hospital wards and one half in coronary care units.

Fatality rates were lower in patients treated at home than those treated in hospital. Such a comparison is valid firstly, if cases were of similar severity (data has been presented indicating that this was so), and secondly, if the delay in receiving care was similar (the median time was about three hours in both groups). A possible source of error was that some of the patients who died suddenly at home and whose deaths were notified to the survey from the coroner's reports or death certificates, had been under the care of general practitioners for several days before, perhaps unrecognised as cases of myocardial infarction and hence not notified as home-treated cases. It could equally be argued that similar cases kept at home who had not died would also modify the figures. A retrospective analysis of the survey data showed that death occurred in twelve such patients who were being treated by general practitioners who had failed to notify them as treated cases, a number insufficient to reverse the better fatality rates for home-treated cases.

The objective criteria we used to assess severity may have been inadequate. The different delay before calling the general practitioner to the two groups has already been discussed. Was this merely a consequence of a patient's reaction to an illness or does it reflect an appropriate response to an illness of different severity, which the general practitioner was able to sense? It is indeed possible that there were subjective differences in severity which were not measurable. All this is highly speculative but clearly we must admit that in spite of the measurements made in this study to assess severity, it is possible that hospital cases may be more severe in a way we could not determine.

What are the implications of these findings and how do they affect the present management of patients with myocardial infarction? It would seem reasonable in the light of our own and other evidence[4] that patients may be left at home if there is a delay of two or three hours before the general practitioner arrives. However, the Teesside study does not resolve the debate as to whether home or hospital is better for the management of cases seen earlier than this. Clearly the present position is unsatisfactory and an attempt should be made to make coronary care facilities available to these patients more quickly. We know that in this survey 50 per cent of patients who died did so suddenly, and a further 21 per cent died within the next two hours. It is difficult to believe that the delay between onset and arrival at a coronary care unit could be shortened sufficiently to reduce fatality significantly using the present system of communication and transportation. During the survey it was estimated that approximately fifteen to thirty patients died in transit between home and hospital.

The basic principle must be that wherever patients are looked after, facilities for the management of the malignant dysrhythmias thought to be the cause of rapid and early deaths should be available to them. This applies particularly in the first two or three hours of care whether at home, work, in the ambulance or in hospital. They must include appropriate analgesic, sedative and anti-dysrhythmic drugs and a defibrillator.

Many patients will be admitted to hospital for social or geographical reasons. There are also well-defined medical criteria for the transfer of patients to hospital. For those admitted to hospital the resuscitation facilities must be provided in the ambulance until the coronary care unit is reached. Some practitioners will prefer to treat their patients at home but they have a duty to provide resuscitative facilities in the very early stages of the illness.

What is the best method of getting resuscitative facilities to the patient as early as possible, regardless of whether the ultimate intention is to admit the patient to hospital or to keep him at home? Our own concept is based on the fact that the general practitioner is usually the first medical attendant to be called. On Teesside 80 per cent of attacks began at home. Only 7 per cent of cases occurred in the street and a further 5 per cent at work and these are the kind of patients who were helped by the ambulance men at Brighton, as described by Dr Chamberlain in Chapter 8. It would seem logical to plan a system which would allow the general practitioner to begin acute resuscitative care in the community. The main objection to providing each general practitioner with a monitor/defibrillator is expense but perhaps more important is the fact that an individual general practitioner does not see sufficient cases to develop the necessary experience. The modern tendency to form group practices, many of which exist in Cleveland, could to some extent overcome these objections. General practitioners must, however, realise that the management of myocardial infarction of recent onset may be a very active process and certainly one which requires constant supervision, very different from the treatment of a stable patient seen three to four hours after the incident.

The system we have evolved in Cleveland is that of a coronary van which transports a hospital-based doctor together with drugs and electrical equipment to a suspected coronary case. Nurses are not involved. The general practitioner may request the van before seeing the patient. He meets the van at the site of the attack and remains responsible for patient management. He decides later whether a case should remain at home or be moved to hospital. In the latter event the patient is taken to hospital by ambulance accompanied by the hospital doctor with the resuscitation equipment from the van. It is obvious that the van, though at present hospital based, could just as well be based in the community and a general practitioner could replace the hospital doctor. This is our eventual objective. We are optimistic that the system should do much to shorten the general practitioner delay factor. The important and longer patient delay before calling for help will not be affected immediately by the system we have outlined. Evidence from Belfast[20] however, shows that the presence of a coronary ambulance in the community, with its attendant publicity, leads to earlier notification by the patient or family and we hope that this will happen locally.

The van we have described requires a clear operational protocol (see Appendix). It is also used by other emergency services — police and ambulance — and by the many large industrial concerns. This covers the

12 per cent of patients whose attack begins at work or in the street. At a later date we intend to consider the possibility that patients could request the van themselves.

We feel that a community approach to the care of patients, involving hospitals and general practitioners is the correct one. Regular training programmes for small groups of general practitioners will be an essential part of this and in any hospital with an established coronary care unit and a nursing training programme in coronary care, this should not be difficult to provide. Long-term education is needed in the community both for patients and for those who look after them.

APPENDIX: CORONARY CARE VAN — GENERAL OPERATING PROTOCOL

1. The Coronary Care Van will be based at the North Tees General Hospital. It will be staffed by the Senior House Officer on Coronary Care Unit duty and will be driven by designated hospital porters. It will cover the North Tees District only.
2. The manner of calling the van will be via the CCU Senior House Officer who will carry a bleep.
3. The designated porter will carry a similar bleep.
4. The coronary van will be equipped with portable resuscitative facilities — drugs, oxygen and monitor/defibrillator.
5. The van is meant to assist the management of a patient who may have suffered an acute myocardial infarction. It is intended to: (i) provide resuscitative facilities for such a patient at an earlier stage in the illness than is at present possible; (ii) supervise the transportation of such a patient to the CCU in hospital if the general practitioner elects for hospital management of the case.
6. The van is *not* intended to be a routine diagnostic service for patients with possible, present or previous ischaemic heart disease. It is also *not* intended to replace the general practitioner at the incident.
7. Rather the basic object is to get resuscitative facilities to a patient in whom there is a reasonable suspicion of a recent ischaemic episode and make these facilities available to the general practitioner.
8. Where the general practitioner receives a call to a patient whose history is highly suggestive of a myocardial infarct during the preceding six hours, it would be appropriate to summon the van as soon as possible (i.e. before seeing the patient). Normally the general practitioner would then meet the van at the patient.

   Where the history and findings suggestive of a myocardial infarct during the preceding six hours are only obtained after the general practitioner has attended the patient, he may if he wishes send for the van but remain with the patient until it arrives

   Where the myocardial infarct has occurred more than six hours but less than forty-eight hours previously the van will not normally be called if the patient is to be kept at home, but the van would be called if the patient needed transporting to hospital, or if complications needing the special facilities arose. In these cases the general practitioner will remain with the patient to meet the van.

The general practitioner should *not* call out the van if he feels his own services are not urgently required as the van is intended to provide facilities additional to and not as a replacement to his own.

9. After initial management the general practitioner may elect to keep the patient at home or send him/her to hospital. If he takes the latter course the patient, hospital doctor and resuscitative equipment will be transferred to the conventional ambulance to cover transportation.

10. If the general practitioner elects to keep the patient at home both he and the van's facilities will remain there for about two hours from the estimated onset of the attack, though this period may have to be curtailed if the van's services are required elsewhere.

11. It is difficult to define precise indications for hospital as opposed to home management of patients with myocardial infarctions, but the following suggestions are made for patients who would need to be transferred to hospital: (i) patients who have had cardiac arrest and resuscitation; (ii) the persistence of malignant or potentially malignant dysrhythmias, e.g. ventricular tachycardia, ventricular ectopics (multiple, R on T, multifocal), heart block; (iii) other medical and social indications at the general practitioner's discretion.

12. Patients with shock or heart failure who are to be transferred to hospital should not be moved until initial treatment is instituted.

13. Training for general practitioners in the emergency management of coronary heart disease, and instruction in the use of resuscitative equipment is available. Any interested practitioner is welcome to arrange this by contracting directly any of the consultant physicians at North Tees General Hospital.

References

1. Armstrong, A. *et al.,* 'Natural History of Acute Coronary Heart Attacks. A Community Study', *British Heart Journal,* 1972, 34, 67-80.
2. Kinlen, L.J., 'Incidence and Presentation of Myocardial Infarction in an English Community', *British Heart Journal,* 1973, 35, 616-22.
3. Pantridge, J.F. and Geddes, J.S., 'A Mobile Intensive Care Unit in the Management of Myocardial Infarction', *Lancet,* 1967, 2, 271.
4. Mather, H.G. *et. al.,* 'Acute Myocardial Infarction: Home and Hospital Treatment', *British Medical Journal,* 1971, 3, 334-8.
5. Smyllie, H.C., Taylor, M.P. and Cuninghame-Green, R.A., '1. Estimating Size of Coronary Care Unit. 2. Delay in Admissions and Survival', *British Medical Journal,* 1972, 1, 31-4.
6. Pedoe, H.T. *et al.,* 'Coronary Heart Attacks in East London', *Lancet,* 1 November 1975, p.833.
7. World Health Organisation, *Hypertension and Coronary Heart Disease: Classification and Criteria for Epidemiological Studies,* Technical Report Series No. 168 (1959).
8. Obratzow, W.P. and Strashesko, N.C., 'Zur Kenntnis der Thrombose der Koronarterien des Herzens', *Z. Klin. Med.,* 1910, 71, 116.
9. Herrick, J.G., 'Clinical Features of Sudden Obstruction of the Coronary Arteries', *Journal of the American Medical Association,* 1912, 59, 2015.
10. Master, A.M., Dack, S. and Jaffe, H.L., 'Premonitory Symptoms of a Coronary Occlusion: A Study of 260 Cases', *Annals of Internal Medicine,* 1941, 14, 1155.
11. Duncan, B. *et al.,* 'Prognosis of New and Worsening Angina Pectoris', *British Medical Journal,* 1976, 1, 981-5.
12. Van Der Does, E. *et al.,* 'Early Warning Symptoms of Acute Myocardial Infarction and Sudden Death', *Hart Bulletin,* 1976, 7, 107-13.
13. Sandler, G. and Pistevos, A., 'Mobile Coronary Care. The Coronary Ambulance', *British Heart Journal,* 1972, 34, 1283-91.
14. Dellipiani, A.W. *et al.,* 'Anxiety after a Heart Attack', *British Heart Journal,* 1976, 38, 752-7.
15. Norris, R.M. *et al.,* 'A New Coronary Prognostic Index', *Lancet,* 1969, i, 274-8.
16. Peel, A.A.F. *et al.,* 'A Coronary Prognostic Index for Grading the Severity of Infarction', *British Heart Journal,* 1962, 24, 745-60.
17. Chapman, B.L., 'Correlation of Mortality Rate and Serum Enzymes in Myocardial Infarction', *British Heart Journal,* 1971, 33, 643-6.
18. Taylor, Lord, 'Poverty, Wealth and Health, or Getting the Dosage Right', *British Medical Journal,* 1975, 4, 207-11.
19. Colling, W.A., 'Home or Hospital Care; Is This the Right Question?', *British Medical Journal,* 1974, 1, 559.
20. Adgey, A.A.J. *et al.,* 'Acute Phase of Myocardial Infarction', *Lancet,* 4 September 1971, pp.501-4.

4 CORONARY CARE IN A NORTH AMERICAN RURAL COMMUNITY: NEWFOUNDLAND

Dr Douglas Black

In Canada the treatment of acute myocardial infarction (AMI) is traditionally hospital based. Very few physicians or patients would be willing to accept home treatment. There have been educational campaigns directed at informing the public about the symptoms of myocardial infarction and the need for the patient to get to hospital as soon as possible. Following demonstration of the effectiveness of the coronary care unit, almost all hospitals have developed them. This applies equally to rural hospitals of less than fifty beds, where it is common to find one or two beds set aside and equipped for cardiac monitoring. These units are staffed by general duty nurses who may have received some extra training, and are supervised by general practitioners who may live a considerable distance from the hospital.

Little effort has been made to evaluate the effectiveness of these small units. Reports in the literature[1-4] suggest that they are effective, but the numbers of patients involved are small and the evidence presented is largely subjective. Cost, in terms of finance and personnel, has not been calculated. Alternative forms of care such as keeping the patient at home or transportation of the patient to a regional hospital in a specially equipped ambulance, have not been evaluated.

Baie Verte

A study was carried out in a practice located on the Baie Verte Peninsula on the north-east coast of Newfoundland, to determine the most appropriate method of caring for patients with AMI in a rural practice. All episodes occurring during a period of seven years were reviewed to determine outcome and adequacy of care. The practice population at the 1971 census was 9,300 scattered in twelve villages. All of the villages are within a radius of 60 km and are connected by gravel roads to the central community where the hospital is located. The nearest large centre with intensive care facilities is 180 km away. The practice area is very well defined and because of the road pattern it is very unlikely that any acutely ill patients left the area without first seeking help from the centrally located hospital.

The population is very stable and there is a very high degree of inter-marriage. The economy is based on two mines, inshore fishing and logging. One investigation performed in this area demonstrated a high incidence of hyperlipidemia in some large families[5] and there are probably other inherited and environmental factors that influence the incidence of disease.

The area is served by a forty-bed hospital built in 1964. which has been staffed by four to six general practitioners who live next to the hospital. For part of the study period there was also a solo general practitioner in a village 60 km from the hospital. It has been the practice of all physicians to admit every patient with suspected AMI to hospital. During most of the study period, no ambulance was available and patients were brought to hospital by private car or taxi. Because of the distance involved, physicians rarely made house calls.

Treatment in hospital consisted largely of bed rest. Digoxin, diuretics, lignocaine and anticoagulants were used only when there were specific indications. A small monitor without an alarm or remote display was available, but unless a special nurse was designated a patient could not be monitored continuously. A defibrillator was also available. During the study period only one patient with an AMI was transferred to another hospital for specialised care.

The Study

The retrospective study covered the seven years from 1 January 1968 to 31 December 1974. All patients admitted during this period and having some form of ischaemic heart disease mentioned in the discharge diagnosis were considered. The records were reviewed, the electrocardiograms re-read and the diagnosis classified according to the World Health Organisation classification.[6, 7] The categories were: Class I (definite), Class II (probable), Class III (possible) and Class VI (insufficient data but no other diagnosis made); those cases which fell into Class IV (no evidence of myocardial infarction) and Class V (no myocardial infarction, another diagnosis made) were not tabulated.

To obtain records on deaths occurring out of hospital, copies of all death certificates made out by doctors in the area were obtained. The records were reviewed on all those cases where there was some mention of heart disease or no other clear diagnosis. Where the clinical chart did not contain enough information the relatives were interviewed. The death was classified as being due to myocardial infarction or other cause according to the criteria given by McWhinney.[8] On only three patients, one dying in hospital and two dying outside, was there autopsy information. Patients from the area who died outside the area were not included and visitors to the area were included. On one visitor in the latter group, who was certified as dying of a myocardial infarction, there were no records available and no relatives could be located.

Results

The results are summarised in Tables 1 and 2. During the seven-year period period there were 217 episodes which fitted the above criteria. Twenty-five of these resulted in deaths outside of hospital. There were 190 patients admitted for care. This would be the number that would require treatment in a specialised unit if such were available and constitutes a patient load of 2.3 per month. Of these patients 92 were in Class III and were subsequently shown not to have had an infarction. They are omitted from further calculations. Of those in Class I, II and VI, 16 died, resulting in a fatality rate of 16.3 per cent.

The age/sex distribution of patients is listed in Table 3. While accurate figures for population by age and sex are not available, it is apparent that this communty has a predominance of the younger age groups, relative to other studied populations. Those under the age of thirty-five constitute 72 per cent of the total population.

Table 4 summarises the cause of death of patients dying in hospital. Of the four patients who died suddenly, possibly of a dysrhythmia, two went into fibrillation before or immediately on arrival at the hospital.

Table 1: Baie Verte Coronary Survey Distribution of Cases by
WHO Classification

Admissions			
	Class I	(Definite)	78
	Class II	(Probable)	19
	Class III	(Possible)	92
	Class VI	(Insufficient Evidence)	1
	Total		190
Other Cases			
	Deaths outside hospital		25
	Undiagnosed sudden deaths in hospital		2
	Total		27
Total Cases			217

Table 2: Fatality and Attack Rates

Hospital Fatality Rate		16.3%
Admissions (Classes I, II & VI)	98	
Deaths (Classes I, II & VI)	16	
Overall Fatality Rate		34.4%
Cases (Classes I, II & VI + deaths)	125	
Total Deaths	43	
Attack Rate (Per 1000 population per year)		1.9%
Cases (Clases I, II & VI + deaths)	125	
Population	9,300	
Mortality Rate (Per 1000 population per year)		0.66%
Total Deaths	43	
Population	9,300	

Table 3: Age-Sex Distribution of Patients

Age	Survivors		In-Hospital Deaths		Out of Hospital Deaths		Sudden Deaths in Hospital	
	M	F	M	F	M	F	M	F
30-39	1							
40-49	6	2	1					
50-59	13	2	3	1	2			
60-69	21	16	1	3	4	3		
70-79	10	5	2	3	9	2		2
80 & over	6		1	1	4	1		

Table 4: Deaths in Hospital (16 Cases)

Average Age	69.5
Causes	
Shock	7
Resistant Failure	3
Pneumonia or Gradual Deterioration	2
Dysrhythmia or Sudden Unexplained Death	4

One other was doing well at seven days post infarction when she died suddenly of what was clinically thought to be pulmonary embolism, and the other was ready for discharge at twenty-one days when he was found dead in bed. Of the others the terminal events were observed and dysrhythmia did not appear to be a significant factor in any of them.

Of those dying out of hospital only two lived for more than one hour after others were aware that they had symptoms. In both of these cases the significance of the symptoms was not recognised until shortly before the patient's death. In all of the other cases the time from onset of symptoms to death was less than the time it would have taken to travel the distance from the hospital to the place of death.

The complications recognised among the survivors are listed in Table 5. The two patients with ventricular fibrillation were successfully resuscitated, one went into fibrillation on the hospital doorstep and the other fibrillated at seven days. The patient with the complete heart block was the one patient who had to be transferred to another hospital.

Table 5: Complications among Survivors (82 Cases)

No complications	44
Cardiac failure	23
Occasional ectopic beats (not treated)	5
Ventricular ectopic beats (treated)	6
Thrombophlebitis and emboli	3
First degree block with bradycardia	1
Complete heart block	1
Ventricular fibrillation	2

Discussion

The attack rate of 1.9 per thousand per year is low when compared to the rate of 4.89 found in the Teesside survey. Other community studies are less easily compared because of differences in criteria used and because complete communities were not studied.[2, 8, 9, 10] Part of this difference is due to the predominance of young people in our population. When the attack rate is calculated for those over the age of thirty-five it is 7.3 in our study and 10.9 in the Teesside survey. The fatality rate of 34.4 per cent would also appear to be low when compared with the 50.5 per cent found in Teesside and similar rates found elsewhere.[8, 11, 12, 13] This rate would be less affected by the population make-up.

In this series, as in others, the majority of deaths occurred before the patient received any medical attention. Because of the distances involved, and because of the short time from onset to death in most cases, it is very unlikely that any form of mobile coronary care would have improved the situation. The delay in seeking help by the patient or the family appeared to be a factor in only two of these deaths.

Among the patients treated in hospital the small number of complications, particularly dysrhythmias, is noteworthy. The number of patients in coronary care units who develop dysrhythmias which require treatment has been reported at 65 per cent or higher.[14, 15] Obviously our rate of 13 per cent is low partly because of the lack of careful monitoring. However, if serious dysrhythmias were missed it would be expected that more patients would have died of dysrthythmias or in a sudden unexplained manner. Only four patients died of what may have been a dysrhythmia, and none occurred during the period that patients are usually kept in coronary care units.

The fatality rate (16.3 per cent) for patients treated in hospital is comparable to that obtained in most coronary care units. The rate is lower if those cases who died in the emergency department are excluded, as is done in many series.

It is difficult to see how any of the deaths could have been prevented by the use of specialised facilities. Ten of the sixteen in-hospital deaths were due to shock or resistant heart failure, a complication that has been little affected by treatment in coronary care units.[1, 2, 16] Intensive monitoring would have been of little use because of the timing of the deaths from dysrhythmia. On the basis of this experience the expenditure in hospital space, staff time and finances to establish a coronary care unit in our hospital can not be justified. Nor is it likely that the transfer of patients to a larger centre would have decreased the fatalities. Some of the patients dying of pneumonia or failure might have been saved by more intensive therapy, but the detrimental effect of the long trip must be set against this possible benefit. In view of the experience at Oxford[17] it is likely that the ill effects of a journey of 180 km would outweigh any possible benefit.

In view of the results of the Bristol study[18] and the experience in Teesside,[19] consideration should be given to treating some patients at home. Home care would be difficult because of the attitudes of the families, the shortage of nurses working in the community and the distances involved. It is possible that in the small hospital some of the benefits of home treatment apply. In a situation without elaborate equipment, with staff that is often known to the patient and where his family can visit freely, there are probably fewer stresses on the patient than in the large specialised hospital some distance from his home. The fact that our patients had so few rhythm disturbances may support the hypothesis that our hospital is less stress producing than a coronary care unit.

Conclusions

It is unlikely that the mortality rate found in this community could have been improved by the use of a mobile coronary care unit, by transferring patients to a larger hospital or by developing a coronary care unit in our hospital. A few deaths might have been prevented by more expert use of drugs and other available forms of treatment which suggests that the emphasis should be on education rather than on equipment.

The results presented here show that treatment in a small hospital may be a satisfactory alternative where home treatment is impractical. They are sufficiently different from those reported from other communities to point out the fallacy of using statistics from different areas to compare the results of forms of treatment. Similarly a community contemplating expenditure on specialised facilities should justify the need on the basis of their own experience and not on the basis of statistics in the literature. The study indicates a need for more community studies to define the incidence and outcome of myocardial infarction in different types of communities in different parts of the world.

Notes

1. Helds, E.H., *Coronary Care in Small Hospitals. The Standish Michigan Experience,* Michigan, W.K. Kellogg Foundation, 1970.
2. Geyman, J.P., 'A Coronary Care Unit in a Small Hospital', *California Medicine,* 1970, 112, 74.
3. Naney, A.P., ' Coronary Care in a Small Rural Hospital', *Journal of the National Medical Association,* 1970, 62, 204.
4. Wickwire, J.C., 'A Coronary Care Unit in a Small Hospital', *Canadian Family Physician,* 1972, 18, 67.
5. Anjilvel, L., 'Familial Hyperlipoproteinemia in an Isolated Part of Newfoundland', *Canadian Medical Association Journal,* 1973, 108, 60.
6. World Health Organisation, *Ischaemic Heart Disease Registers,* Report of Fourth Working Group, Copenhagen, July 1970.

7. World Health Organisation, *Ischaemic Heart Disease Registers,* Report of Working Group, Copenhagen, May 1968.
8. McWhinney, I.R., 'Incidence of Ischaemic Heart Disease in a Country Town Group Practice', *Lancet,* 1968, II, 342.
9. Armstrong, A. *et al.,* 'Natural History of Acute Coronary Heart Attacks. A Community Study', *British Heart Journal,* 1972, 34, 67.
10. Smyllie, H.C., Taylor, M.P. and Cuninghame-Green, R.A., 'Acute Myocardial Infarction in Doncaster. I. Estimating Size of Coronary Care Unit', *British Medical Journal,* 1972, 1, 31.
11. Sleet, R.A., 'Report of 24 Cases of Myocardial Infarction Treated at Home', *British Medical Journal,* 1968, 4, 675.
12. Fry, J. and Dillane, J.B., 'Acute Coronary Deaths', *Journal of the Royal College of General Practitioners,* 1967, 14, 44.
13. Fulton, M.B., Julian, D.G. and Oliver, M.F., 'Sudden Death and Myocardial Infarction', *Circulation,* 1969, 39 and 40, suppl.4, 182.
14. MacMillan, R.L. and Brown, K.W.G., 'Comparison of the Effects of Treatment of Acute Myocardial Infarction in a Coronary Care Unit and on a General Medical Ward', *Canadian Medical Association Journal,* 1971, 105, 1037.
15. Lown, B. and Selzer, A., 'Controversies in Cardiology: The Coronary Care Unit', *American Journal of Cardiology,* 1968, 22, 597.
16. Yu, P.N. *et al.,* 'Resources for the Optimal Care of Patients with Acute Myocardial Infarction', Study Group on Coronary Heart Disease, *Circulation,* 1971, 43, A-171-83.
17. Kinlen, L.J., 'Incidence and Presentation of Myocardial Infarction in an English Community', *British Heart Journal,* 1973, 35, 616-22.
18. Mather, H.G. *et al.,* 'Acute Myocardial Infarction: Home and Hospital Treatment', *British Medical Journal,* 1971, 3, 334.
19. Colling, W.A., 'Teesside Coronary Survey: An Epidemiological Study of Acute Attacks of Myocardial Infarction', *British Medical Journal,* 1976, 2, 1169-72.

PART TWO   GIVING CORONARY CARE

5 HOME AND HOSPITAL CARE: THE NOTTINGHAM EXPERIMENT

Dr David Hill

The Nottingham Home or Hospital Study is in progress at the present time. Its object is to allocate patients with suspected myocardial infarction and without apparent complications to home or hospital management, on a random basis, and to assess the effects of the two forms of management on fatality.

The Problem

There has been much debate over the past few years about the relative values of coronary care units and coronary ambulances manned by doctors or specially trained ambulancemen. Much of the evidence available on the subject of home management is uncoordinated or retrospective. The results of the only controlled trial[1] of home or hospital management of myocardial infarction have never been accepted by the medical community in general for various reasons. Apart from this trial, the evidence is mostly circumstantial and does little to help the doctor faced with the problem of what to do with a patient suffering from a suspected myocardial infarction in his home. As most such cases present to the health services in this manner in Britain, it is therefore the general practitioner who has to make the choice of how to manage such a patient. The decision must often be made on the patient's history, as further information will not be available until later. The decision of how to manage such a patient is made on the basis of the doctor's experience, and his knowledge of the local situation.

The Evidence

There is no doubt that many patients have been treated (knowingly or unknowingly) at home for their myocardial infarction, with apparent success. In a recent survey in Nottingham,[2] 305 practitioners were asked: 'How would you manage a forty-five-year-old man with a history typical of myocardial infarction, living in good social circumstances?' Of the 179 practitioners who gave an unqualified answer, 39 per cent said that they would manage the patient at home. There was a higher preference for home management in those practitioners who qualified before 1960.

There is increasing evidence that in this country at least, patients with suggestive symptoms exclude themselves from early help by not calling their own doctor until after the maximum danger period has passed. During 1974-5, in 1,250 consecutive patients with suspected myocardial infarction transported to the Nottingham hospitals,[3] an ambulance had been called in only 8 per cent of cases by a general practitioner within thirty minutes from the onset of symptoms (Figure 1). In contrast, when the ambulance was called by a relative, 50 per cent of patients had requested help in the same period of time. It seems reasonable, therefore, that most of the general practitioner cases do not stand to benefit from hospital-based coronary care services, whether mobile or static, by the time they are first seen.

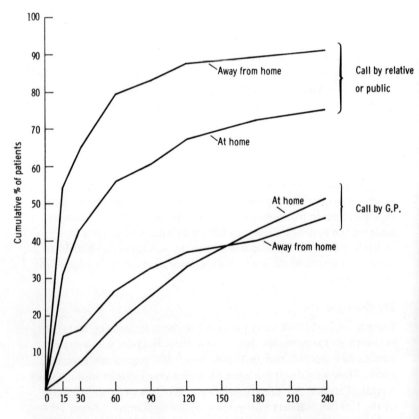

Figure 1   Duration of symptoms before ambulance call in the different groups of patients

Various community surveys are described elsewhere in this book; most, especially the Teesside survey,[4] lend strength to the idea that the fatality rate of cases left at home is at least no worse than that of the hospitalised group. The only controlled trial of home or hospital care for patients with suspected myocardial infarction was that of Mather and colleagues in the south-west of England, published in 1971 and 1976.[1] The results of this trial have been hotly debated, in this book and elsewhere. Although the mortality of the group randomly allocated to home care was significantly less than that of the random hospital group, these results have never gained general acceptance, principally because of the low randomisation rate (28 per cent) which the investigators achieved. The argument of home versus hospital care for myocardial infarction thus continues to rage.

The Nottingham Study

It was with this background that a Department of Health and Social Security support grant was obtained to make a randomised study of home and hospital care, which began in 1973. General practitioners in specific areas in and around Nottingham notify a hospital-based team (a Senior House Officer and a CCU-trained nurse) when they receive a call which leads them to believe that the patient may have a myocardial infarction. The team then goes to the patient's home in a specially equipped estate car. Once at the house, any necessary emergency treatment is given and arrangements are made for those patients who need urgent hospital treatment to be admitted. Those patients who are unsuitable for trial purposes are electively managed in a manner appropriate to their condition, and fall broadly into the following groups:

1. Patients whose symptoms do not lead the team to suspect a myocardial infarction.
2. Patients with suspected myocardial infarction but who: (i) are successfully resuscitated from a cardiorespiratory arrest; (ii) have complications thought to require hospital treatment (e.g. complete heart block); (iii) have co-incidental disease requiring hospital treatment; (iv) are socially unsuitable to be managed at home; this group also includes those who demand either home or hospital treatment (see Figure 2).

For the remainder, provided that the suspicion of myocardial infarction persists, the team stays in the house for two hours, monitoring and

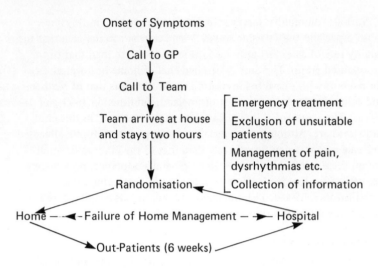

Figure 2   Randomisation of Cases: Flow chart of patients coming under care.

treating any pain, dysrhythmias, etc. At the end of that time a sealed
envelope, containing a random card allocating the patient to home or
hospital treatment, is opened. The patient is then managed according
to the course indicated on the card. Evidence is collected according
to a set plan in both groups, and all patients, except those who die,
are seen in the out-patient clinic six weeks after the event. Patients in
the randomised home group, who subsequently require admission for
either medical or social reasons, are designated 'home failures' but
remain in their original groups for the purpose of classification.

The Results

At the time of writing, no meaningful fatality results are available.
However, a broad analysis of the first 300 calls is useful, as it has
important implications for any domiciliary services. Of the first 300
calls, there were 201 cases of suspected myocardial infarction. The
remainder consisted of assorted cardiovascular emergencies (16), other
chest pain (55), and other calls with good intent (28). Of the 201 cases
of suspected myocardial infarction, 153 (76 per cent) were considered
eligible for the trial and were randomly allocated to the treatment
groups. The remainder (48) were excluded on the grounds discussed

above. This randomisation rate is nearly three times that of the Bristol and south-west trial, and has not changed since the Nottingham trial began.

The calling times of patients in relation to their onset of symptoms have been analysed, and again show the significant element of patient induced delay. Only 23 per cent of patients had requested any help within thirty minutes of the onset of symptoms. This reflects the difficulties of providing an effective domiciliary service for cases of suspected myocardial infarction called by a general practitioner.

Finally, as a measure of the impact of such a service on fatality rates, the number of resuscitations has been analysed. During the first 300 calls, four patients were successfully resuscitated in their homes from ventricular fibrillation. All four were alive and apparently well on admission to hospital, but one died in the hospital coronary care unit, and two more died during the remainder of their hospital admission. There was thus one survivor from domiciliary resuscitation to come to out-patients six weeks after the event. He has since died.

It is concluded from these facts, and from other studies, that hospital-based domiciliary services called by general practitioners to cases of suspected myocardial infarction are unlikely to make a major contribution to the lowering of community mortality. Final results of this study should be available during 1977.

References

1. Mather, H.G. *et al.,* 'Acute Myocardial Infarction: Home and Hospital Treatment', *British Medical Journal,* 1971, 3, 334-8.
2. Hampton, J.R., Morris, G.K. and Mason, C., 'Survey of General Practitioners' Attitudes to Management of Patients with Heart Attacks', *British Medical Journal,* 1975, 4, 146-8.
3. Hill, J.D. and Hampton, J.R., 'Importance of Patient Selection in Evaluating a Cardiac Ambulance Service', *British Medical Journal,* 1976, 1, 201-3.
4. Colling, W.A. *et al.,* 'Teesside Coronary Survey: An Epidemiological Study of Acute Attacks of Myocardial Infarction', *British Medical Journal,* 1976, 2, 1169-72.

6

WHAT DOES INTENSIVE CARE ACHIEVE?

Professor D.G. Julian

In order to evaluate the achievements and limitations of intensive care it is necessary to consider its place in relation to acute heart attacks to both in the community and in hospital.

In the community studies from Edinburgh and Belfast,[1, 2] 50 per cent of deaths occurred within the first two hours. There was still a considerable number of deaths throughout the first day but during the rest of the month subsequent to onset there were comparatively few. It is useful to look at this another way. If one sees a patient at the moment he has his heart attack, that patient has a 40 to 50 per cent chance of dying within the next month. If one waited an hour before seeing him he would have a 28 per cent chance of dying. Thus the fatality will differ depending on the time a patient is seen. The later one sees patients, the better the results will appear to be. The quicker that patients are admitted to hospital the higher the hospital mortality will tend to be. If patients who are admitted early are found to have a low death rate then one is probably doing something good.

It was long ago apparent that ventricular fibrillation (VF) was the predominant cause of death in patients who reached hospital in the early phase of acute myocardial infarction (AMI) and that a high proportion of these deaths were taking place very early indeed. We now know from the experience of mobile coronary care units (MCCU) everywhere that the overwhelming cause of death in the first hour is VF. Prior to intensive coronary care one third of deaths in hospitalised patients were due to VF; shock, failure, ventricular rupture and pulmonary embolism were responsible for the remainder. It was commonplace in those days for patients in 'good condition' to die suddenly; this has become a rarity when there is intensive care but doubts as to its value continue.

Importance of Relief of Pain

What can intensive care really do? What are the therapeutic measures we should be involved in both outside and inside hospital? It is not enough to say that we should get an ambulance to the patient — that is of no use whatsoever if you do not do anything useful when you have got it there. Pain relief, although it might not be called intensive care, is of immense importance. This is worth stressing because we have found that many general practitioners, including those who send their patients into hospital very quickly, send them in without relieving their pain. This is a wrong practice both on humanitarian grounds and because the pain has a highly undesirable effect — it increases the autonomic reaction to the infarction, and probably encourages the development of dysrhythmias and shock. A lot of practitioners are afraid of giving morphine or other potent analgesics because they think the patient might have a perforated ulcer and they would be in terrible trouble with the surgeons. It is surely better to risk giving morphine inappropriately to an ulcer than not to give it to an infarct.

Morphine or diamorphine (heroin) should be given in quite large doses, intravenously in the first place. Obviously there are patients for whom this treatment may be inappropriate, those with respiratory disease for example. Those with a slow heart rate should certainly be protected with atropine, given with or before morphine, and we like to give trifluoperazine (stelazine) or cyclizine (valoid) together with morphine to prevent vomiting. Diamorphine is certainly a very effective drug but it can deteriorate on the shelf and one needs to make sure that it is reasonably fresh. Nitrous oxide (as 'Entonox') is a useful analgesic, particularly in patients to whom one does not want to give morphine or who have failed to respond to morphine. It has the advantage that ambulance drivers can give it. The other analgesics — particularly pethidine — are not particularly desirable because they can lead to hypotension and tachycardia. Of course, morphine can also lead to hypotension but usually one can protect the patient from it by giving atropine or cyclizine.

Bradycardia

One of the problems which occurs very early in a substantial proportion of patients with infarction is bradycardia — most commonly sinus bradycardia. There has been a lot of controversy about the potential hazard of a slow heart rate — some authorities have said it is desirable and others have said it is dangerous. Both are right; it depends on the timing of the bradycardia and on the associated features. Bradycardia twenty-four hours after infarction is associated with a good prognosis; the presence of bradycardia means that there is not the tachycardia associated with heart failure. On the other hand, bradycardia in the first hour is often accompanied by hypotension or dysrhythmia; if these are present one should correct the rate.

As an example, we had a patient with sinus bradycardia at 50/min.

seen about twenty minutes after the onset by the MCCU in Edinburgh, in whom we were unable to record the blood pressure (Figure 1 (a)). The woman was obviously very sick — the people who attended her thought she was moribund — but she was given 0.6 mg atropine intravenously. There was immediate improvement — her heart rate accelerated to 80/min. and her blood pressure rose to 150/90 and one would not have known she had a heart attack (Figure 1 b). This is not an uncommon event and striking changes may be seen in the ECG when the rate is corrected.

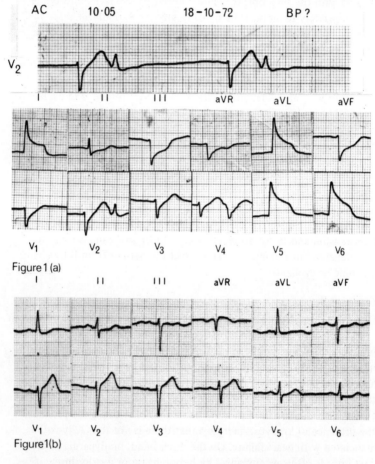

Figure 1 (a)

Figure 1(b)

Figure 1   (a) Rhythm strip in patient with unrecordable blood pressure, and
   12-lead ECG. (b) 12-lead ECG of same patient 20 minutes after atropine. The
   heart rate has increased to 80/min. with the disappearance of ST segment
   changes.

Heart Block

The other cause of bradycardia is heart block; its significance also depends on the circumstances. Heart block, like sinus bradycardia, is fairly common in the early acute phase and at this time is similarly related to excessive parasympathetic tone and may be readily treated by atropine.

We had a patient with complete heart block and a ventricular rate of 20-30. The changes of inferior infarction were present, with extreme ST elevation (Figure 2). The blood pressure was unrecordable. He was treated with intravenous atropine and within five minutes his heart rate had accelerated, and normal rhythm and blood pressure had been restored. The ST segments became almost normal. By the next day, the ECG changes were minimal.

These two cases demonstrate the importance in some cases of treating slow rhythms in the early phase perhaps preventing the area of infarction enlarging.

Many cases of heart block seen in hospital develop several hours after admission; these usually do not respond to atropine. If the infarct is inferior, the heart block will frequently resolve spontaneously within a few hours or a few days. There may be a period when the patient is liable to Stokes-Adams attacks and to heart failure. Such patients undoubtedly appear to benefit from pacing but most will survive without it – the number actually saved by pacing is small. At the other end of the spectrum are those with heart block and anterior infarction. To get heart block with anterior infarction one must have massive damage involving the septum; these patients are very likely to die whatever one does. Pacing may temporarily save their lives but in the long term the prognosis is bad. In summary, pacing helps heart block both in inferior and anterior infarcts but only a small proportion of cases are salvaged because of it.

Ventricular Dysrhythmias

Ventricular dysrhythmias have become a more difficult problem in recent years. The traditional concern of CCUs is that patients who have certain ventricular dysrhythmias are at risk from VF and of course VF is the complication one is most concerned to prevent. Certain sorts of ventricular dysrhythmias appear particularly predictive of VF, – R on T ectopic beats (Figure 3), frequent ectopic beats, those occurring in runs of two or three, those with varying patterns and ventricular tachycardia. By careful and continuous monitoring we now

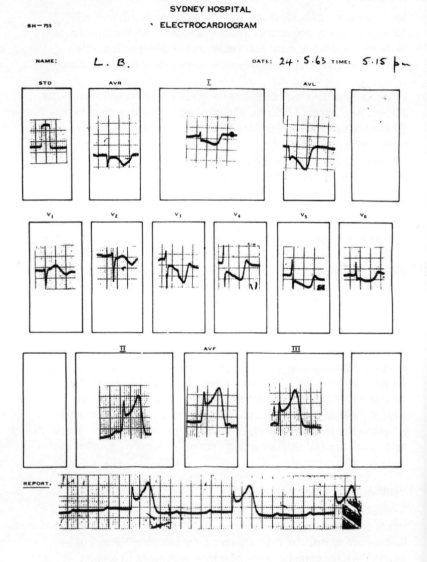

Figure 2   12-lead ECG of patient and (below) a rhythm strip of patient with inferior myocardial infarction. There is complete heart block with a ventricular rate of 30/min.

know that ventricular dysrhythmias are extremely common and that in many cases they do not go on to VF. Furthermore, we know that many cases of VF have had no prior 'warning' dysrhythmia. This obviously has important implications. If certain types of ventricular dysrhythmia are to be detected then enormous resources must be devoted to the task. It has been shown that even in a good CCU many of these ventricular dysrhythmias are missed and to recognise them reliably you need a computer. On the other hand, as VF can happen out of the blue — why bother? Or, why not try to prevent VF by treating everybody?

For the time being I think we should assume that certain ventricular dysrhythmias are dangerous and I would particularly emphasise R on T ectopic beats, runs of two or more ectopic beats, and those with varying shapes. If one finds these sorts of dysrhythmia then one should treat them with intravenous lignocaine. Dosage has also been a problem — there is no doubt that in the past we have given too little. One should start between 50 and 100 mg intravenously — about 75 mg for the average-sized person. It is important not to give it too fast as many patients can get dizzy or even confused. The manufacturers suggest that you then give 2-4 mg per minute by intravenous infusion. This is potentially dangerous (at least 4 mg a minute is) but on the other hand if you start at 2 mg a minute it takes some time before you get adequate control of the rhythm. Ideally what one should do is to start with 4 mg a minute for about fifteen minutes and then reduce the rate to 2 mg a minute. An alternative possibility as far as general practice is concerned is to give a combination of lignocaine 75 mg intravenously together with 300 mg intramuscularly into the deltoid.

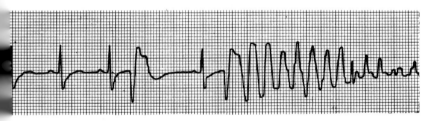

Figure 3   R on T ectopic beats, the second of which initiates ventricular fibrillation

If a doctor is with a patient when he goes into VF and he had a defibrillator he should not start by giving him closed chest massage and ventilation — he should defibrillate him at once. If this is not effective or a defibrillator is not available then other methods must be used. In defibrillating VF one does not necessarily need large energies — 200 Joules is the right dose to start with. We did a number of experiments trying different doses: 100 Joules fails too frequently for comfort but 200 Joules works in nearly all cases.

How Valuable Is Intensive Care?

Does intensive care really do any good at all? The figures from Hofvendahl in Stockholm are the most important as far as hospital CCUs are concerned.[3] This was the nearest to a controlled trial that has been carried out in a hospital CCU. At the time, there was an inadequate number of beds for all patients, so patients were allocated to the CCU and general ward, depending only on bed availability. The result was a very substantial difference between ward and CCU — the fatality rate was halved in the CCU. Furthermore, this difference was maintained after thirty-six months. This was purely a hospital study; there has been no satisfactory controlled study comparing home and hospital or home and CCU.

We are all now well aware of the limited amount a hospital CCU can do about the overall mortality in the community, but I personally believe that it is impossible not to think that the successful treatment of VF has not affected mortality. The fact that the statisticians cannot prove it should not bother us — there are a lot of things they cannot find. If one reduces overall mortality by 3 or 5 per cent they will not be able to demonstrate it, but 3 or 5 per cent of the 100,000 people dying a year is a significant number of people in human terms if not statistically.

Delay in Receiving Care

If we accept the value of intensive care in the early stages of infarction, it is important that it should be available as soon as possible. But experience shows that long intervals usually occur between onset and treatment. In the Edinburgh community study the median time which a patient took to contact his GP was 1 hour 44 minutes. This figure needs some elaboration because this is the actual time it took for the general practitioner to receive the call. If his telephone was engaged or if he was out on a call or if he could not be reached then that time delay was included. Furthermore, if the patient had difficulty in reaching a telephone because the local one had been ruined by vandals, that time was also included; so this figure is not all the patient's or his relatives' fault. It took an average of 51 minutes from the receipt of the call by the general practitioner to the general practitioner arriving at the patient's home. The general practitioner on average took 33 minutes after having arrived in the home to call an ambulance; it took 10 minutes to get hold of the ambulance and a further 20 minutes for the ambulance to arrive. The journey from home to hospital took 21 minutes and 29 minutes were spent lingering in the casualty department — a total of 4 hours 28 minutes. The figures from European centres vary enormously — the mean figure in Helsinki is one hour, the mean figure in Prague is fifteen hours! This is partly a matter of definitions and interpretations and partly a matter of the organisation of health services. The introduction of a MCCU in Edinburgh reduced the median time from about 4½ hours to about 2 hours, and the number of patients receiving intensive care within 1 hour rose from 2 to 25 per cent.

Education of Patients

We have been interested to find out whether by education of patients we could get them to call their doctor earlier, because the biggest delay is the time it takes the patient to call the doctor. In other countries a great deal of time and money has been spent on educating patients and the public to call the doctor without delay.

I thought we should first analyse why some people call their doctor early and others call him late. I first did an analysis on cardiologists who had coronaries because I assumed they were intelligent and educated. In fact the median time for the cardiologist to call his doctor was forty-eight hours! Then Dr Vetter in Edinburgh looked at the patients who called their doctors early to see if they were more apprehensive or whether they had had a previous infarction, previous angina or whatever. There was only one outstanding factor — the suddenness of the onset of the symptoms. If the patient fainted or felt weak or if he collapsed in the street then a doctor was called quickly. If he was suddenly afflicted by the most intense pain out of the blue, he called a doctor without delay. If, on the other hand, he had a stuttering sort of pain, particularly if he had had angina before, he was not so quick to call the doctor. The pain caused by an infarction varies greatly, so the nature of the onset is the thing which really seems to determine how the patient behaves, and how everyone else behaves — the delays right down the line are affected by the nature of the attack.

Thus, the diagnostic delay — the time the doctor takes to make up his mind what to do — is affected. If a man has collapsed or is in severe pain the doctor gets on with things without waiting to make a precise diagnosis. If the pain is indefinite he takes longer. When we look at figures from different centres and the comparisons between home and hospital, we must not assume that those who call their doctors early are necessarily more severe or less severe than the others — we do not know the prognosis of these two groups. For example, in interpreting the results from the south-west of England,[4, 5] it is interesting to note that the median time for the general practitioner first seeing the patient was 4 hours compared with 3 hours in Teesside[6] and 2½ hours in Edinburgh.[1] This may well play an important part in the results. If the general practitioner gets there late it is not going to make much difference what he does.

Notes

1. Armstrong, A. *et al.,* 'Natural History of Unstable Angina', *Lancet,* 1972, 1, 860.
2. McNeilly, R.H. and Pemberton, J., 'Duration of Last Attack in 998 Fatal Cases of Coronary Artery Disease and Its Relation to Possible Cardiac Resuscitation', *British Medical Journal,* 1968, 3, 139.
3. Hofvendahl, S., 'Influence of Treatment in a Coronary Care Unit on Prognosis in Acute Myocardial Infarction', *Acta Medica Scandanavica,* 1971, Suppl.519.
4. Mather, H.G. *et al.,* 'Acute Myocardial Infarction: Home and Hospital Treatment', *British Medical Journal,* 1971, 3, 334-8.
5. Mather, H.G. *et al.,* 'Myocardial Infarction. A Comparison between Home and Hospital Care for Patients', *British Medical Journal,* 1976, 1, 925-9.
6. Colling, W.A. *et al.,* 'Teesside Coronary Survey: An Epidemiological Study of Acute Attacks of Myocardial Infarction in a Large Urban Community', *British Medical Journal,* 1976, 2, 1169-72.

7 PRE-HOSPITAL CORONARY CARE WITH A MOBILE UNIT

Dr Jennifer Adgey

There are some 55,000 premature deaths from acute myocardial infarction in Great Britain every year (Table 1). Sixty-three per cent of deaths from acute myocardial infarction among males aged fifty or less occur within one hour[1] and among patients of both sexes under the age of sixty-five with an initial coronary attack 61 per cent of the deaths occur within that time[2] (Table 2). We have shown that the mechanism of death is ventricular fibrillation in more than 90 per cent of those who die suddenly.[3, 4]

Table 1: Annual Deaths from Acute Myocardial Infarction (Less than 70 Years)

	1968	1969	1970	1971	1972
England and Wales	45,826	46,934	46,638	46,909	49,050
Scotland	6,590	6,727	6,756	6,792	7,125
N. Ireland	1,488	1,445	1,577	1,489	1,627
Total	53,904	55,106	54,971	55,190	57,802

Table 2: Deaths within 1 Hour of the Onset of the Coronary Attack

	Age Groups	Sex	Period from Onset	Deaths within 1 Hour
Seattle (Bainton & Peterson, 1963)	50 and <	M.	14 Days	63%
Belfast (McNeilly & Pemberton, 1968)	All Ages	M. & F.	4 Weeks	41%
Framingham (Gordon & Kannel, 1971)	<65	M. & F.	30 Days	61%
Edinburgh (Armstrong et al., 1972)	<70	M. & F.	4 Weeks	45%

Belfast Mobile Coronary Care Unit

In view of the high incidence of early sudden death, a mobile coronary care unit was initiated in Belfast in January 1966. The personnel consists of a junior doctor and a nurse or medical student. They carry to the site of the attack, e.g. the patient's home, a battery-operated direct current defibrillator, oxygen, a battery-operated monitoring oscilloscope tape recorder, drugs and intravenous solutions required to stabilise the cardiac rhythm (Figure 1). All the equipment is portable. The hardware is robust and, as far as possible, foolproof. Since the apparatus must, on occasions, be carried some distance and possibly in haste up several flights of stairs, the monitoring equipment and defibrillator are light and compact. It is unnecessary to use clumsy, expensive and heavy defibrillators since small models are available.

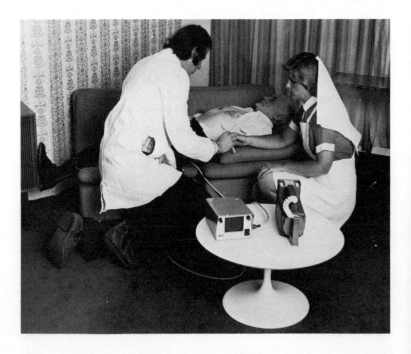

Figure 1   Initiation of monitoring and therapy in the patient's home

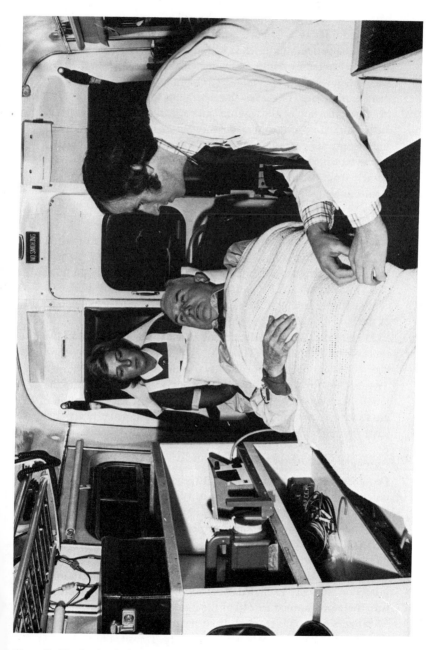

Figure 2 Monitoring during transport

When the team reaches the patient he will be under the same intensive care conditions as obtain in a hospital coronary care unit. Fifty per cent of the patients are reached within ten minutes of receipt of the call from the family doctor or lay individual and nearly three quarters are reached within fifteen minutes. When the mobile team arrives, therapy is initiated or that of the general practitioner continued. Pain relief, stabilisation of the rhythm and correction of the autonomic disturbance are considered mandatory before movement. Monitoring and therapy are continued during transport (Figure 2). Haste or fuss during transport is most carefully avoided. The patient is transferred directly from the ambulance to the hospital coronary care unit, monitoring continuing during this transfer.

Primary Ventricular Fibrillation

Since clinical observation of patients seen within one hour of the onset of myocardial infarction might yield information regarding the factors precipitating ventricular fibrillation, a detailed prospective study was made of 294 patients. From the time of the initial observation continuous recording of the electrocardiogram and frequent estimations of the blood pressure were made.

Primary ventricular fibrillation occurred at some time in 55 (19 per cent) of the 294 patients (Figure 3). Forty-one (75 per cent) of the 55 had ventricular fibrillation within two hours of the onset of symptoms. Twenty-three of the fifty-five had ventricular fibrillation before the mobile team arrived. Those who developed ventricular fibrillation often did so without warning dysrhythmias or despite apparently adequate antiarrhythmic therapy.

Autonomic Disturbance

Documentation of the autonomic disturbance at the time of the initial observation was attempted. Assessment of autonomic disturbance was impossible in those patients who presented with ventricular fibrillation, ventricular tachycardia or supraventricular dysrhythmias, and in those who had been on digitalis or beta-blocking agents prior to the onset of infarction. Patients with a known history of hypertension and those with left bundle branch block or combined anterior and posterior infarction were also excluded. Analysis of the autonomic disturbance was, therefore, limited to 240 of the 294 patients.

Patients with sinus tachycardia at the initial examination were considered to have sympathetic overactivity. Transient hypertension (blood pressure 160/100 mm Hg or greater) in the absence of sinus

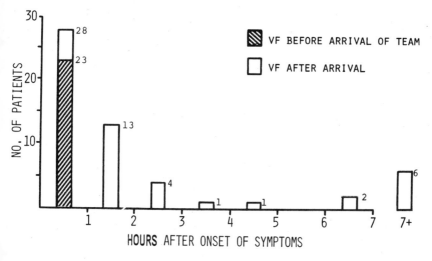

Figure 3   Incidence of primary ventricular fibrillation in 294 patients seen within 1 hour

tachycardia was regarded as evidence of sympathetic overactivity. Patients with sinus bradycardia or atrio-ventricular block (second degree or complete) were considered to show parasympathetic overactivity. Transient hypertension (systolic blood pressure 100 mm Hg or less) in the absence of bradycardia was also regarded as evidence of parasympathetic overactivity.

Eighty-nine of the 240 patients were seen within thirty minutes. Only fifteen (17 per cent) of the eighty-nine had a normal heart rate and normal blood pressure when first seen (Figure 4). Over one third showed evidence of sympathetic overactivity. Parasympathetic overactivity was present in almost half of the patients. The systolic blood pressure at the initial examination was not greater than 80 mm Hg in nearly one quarter of the patients. Forty-seven per cent of the patients with bradyarrhythmia had a systolic blood pressure not greater than 80 mm Hg. Eight per cent of all patients seen within thirty minutes

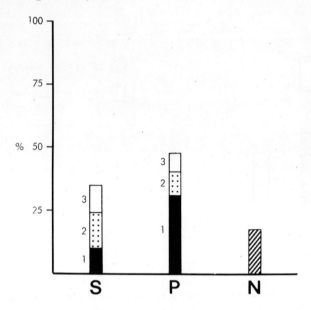

Figure 4   Evidence of autonomic disturbance in 89 patients seen within 30 minutes

S = sympathetic overactivity	P = parasympathetic overactivity
S1 = sinus tachycardia with hypertension	P1 = bradyarrhythmia with hypotension
S2 = sinus tachycardia	P2 = bradyarrhythmia
S3 = transient hypertension	P3 = transient hypotension

N = normal heart rate and blood pressure

had complete atrio-ventricular block; none of these had a systolic blood pressure greater than 80 mm Hg.

The incidence of autonomic disturbance was related to the site of infarction (Figure 5). Parasympathetic overactivity occurred more frequently in association with posterior infarction (p < 0.001).

Of the 240 patients, 151 were seen within the second half of the first hour. The incidence of autonomic disturbance was significantly lower (p < 0.001) among these than among the patients seen within thirty minutes (Figure 6). Eighty-three per cent of the patients seen within thirty minutes showed evidence of autonomic disturbance whereas only 56 per cent of those seen within the second half of the first hour showed this disturbance at the initial observation.

Various mechanisms have been suggested to account for the early

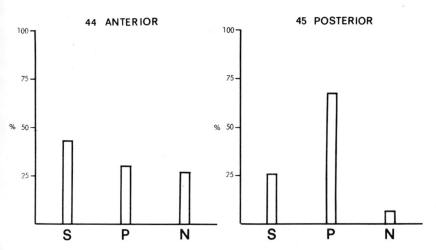

Figure 5   Autonomic disturbance among patients seen within 30 minutes:
44 with anterior infarction and 45 with posterior infarction

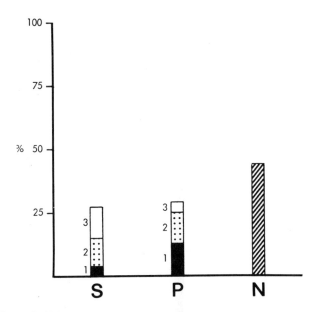

Figure 6   Evidence of autonomic disturbance in 151 patients seen within the
second half of the first hour. Key as for Figure 4

bradycardia and hypotension. More than a century ago Von Bezold
described in animals a cardiogenic reflex precipitating bradycardia and
hypotension.[5] Stimulation of the vagal neuroreceptors in the region of
the coronary sinus and atrio-ventricular node may produce the human
counterpart of the Von Bezold-Jarisch reflex.[6] The anatomical
distribution of these vagal receptors may be the reason for the greater
frequency of parasympathetic overactivity in patients with posterior
infarction. When patients with previous infarction, which may have
interfered with the vagal receptors, were excluded, evidence of
parasympathetic overactivity was almost invariable among patients
with posterior infarction seen within thirty minutes (Figure 7). While
reflex vagal overactivity may produce atrio-ventricular block, the effect
of ischaemia on the atrio-ventricular node may be an accentuating
factor. Occlusion of the right coronary artery usually occurs distal to
the origin of the sinus node artery and proximal to the origin of the
artery to the atrio-ventricular node. One of the effects of ischaemia
may be inhibition of cholinesterase activity and an accumulation of
acetylcholine in the region of the atrio-ventricular node.[7] Larger
amounts of atropine are usually required for the correction of
atrio-ventricular block than for the correction of sinus bradycardia.[8]

Effects of Parasympathetic Overactivity

There are two aspects of the problem regarding the importance of
bradycardia following acute myocardial infarction: (1) the effects of
the slow heart rate on the ischaemic zone surrounding the infarct and
(2) the relationship of bradycardia to ventricular dysrhythmias.

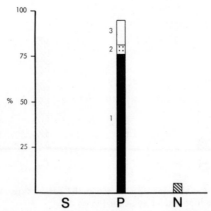

Figure 7   Autonomic disturbance among 21 patients with posterior infarction
seen within 30 minutes (first infarction). Key as for Figure 4

The effect of bradycardia on the ischaemic zone surrounding the infarct will depend on the magnitude of the fall in blood pressure that accompanies the slow heart rate. In almost half the patients with bradycardia the systolic blood pressure was not over 80 mm Hg. Reduction in the heart rate in the patient with myocardial infarction may not be compensated for by an increase in stroke volume. Thus, a fall in blood pressure and cardiac output results. The hypotension that accompanies early bradycardia may also be related to the known loss of atrial transport function which results from vagal stimulation even in the absence of atrio-ventricular block.[9] In addition, vagal overactivity exerts a negative inotropic effect on the ventricle.[10, 11] The hypotension resulting from bradycardia is likely to lead to extension of the initial area of infarction and to an increased incidence of shock and pump failure.[12]

Malignant ectopic beats may appear when the heart rate slows (Figure 8). Furthermore, ectopics in the presence of a slow heart rate may be abolished by increasing the rate. Since the incidence of bradycardia and the incidence of ventricular fibrillation are both high immediately after the onset of acute myocardial infarction, it has been suggested that bradycardia may be a precursor of ventricular fibrillation and an important factor in the early high fatality from acute myocardial infarction.[8] On the other hand, it has been reported that hospitalised patients who show sinus bradycardia have a good prognosis.[13, 14, 15] The difference may be related to the time after the onset of symptoms at which bradycardia occurs. Bradycardia and hypotension appearing immediately after the onset of infarction may differ significantly from bradycardia occurring later in hospital. Certainly, the sudden development of bradycardia in the acute phase of myocardial infarction may lead to ventricular tachycardia (Figure 9) or ventricular fibrillation (Figure 10). Even when the overall heart rate is within the normal range, the occasional prolonged R-R interval may be dangerous (Figure 11).

Effects of Sympathetic Overactivity

Observations within thirty minutes indicate that sympathetic overactivity is present in 35 per cent of patients with myocardial infarction and in a further 8 per cent sympathetic overactivity may be unmasked by the correction of vagal overactivity. It is of interest that when patients are observed immediately after the onset of spontaneously occurring angina pectoris, evidence suggesting sympathetic overactivity is invariable.[16] Acute myocardial infarction is accompanied by an immediate rise in blood catecholamines.[17-20]

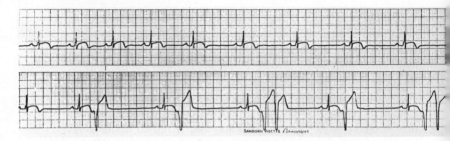

Figure 8 Continuous record: ventricular ectopics appear when the rate slows
from 62 to 45

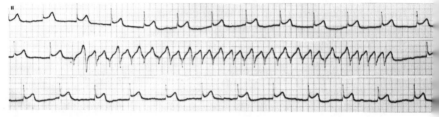

Figure 9 Acute posterior infarct, lead 2. Nodel bradycardia with unrecordable
blood pressure and the sudden appearance of self-terminating ventricular
tachycardia/ventricular flutter (continuous record in patient's home)

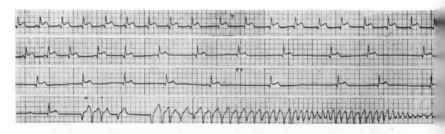

Figure 10 Acute myocardial infarction, lead 2. Sudden onset of sinus
bradycardia with hypotension (systolic blood pressure 80 mm Hg) and the
appearance of ventricular fibrillation (continuous record in patient's home)

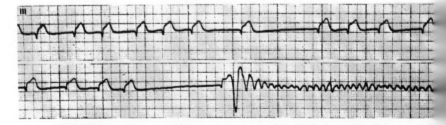

Figure 11 Continuous record during the second hour after the onset of acute
posterior infarction. Atrial fibrillation, ventricular rate 62 per minute. An R
on T ventricular ectopic leading to ventricular fibrillation occurred following
a prolonged R-R interval

This response probably results from neurogenic reflexes arising from the infarcted and contiguous areas.[21, 22] While adrenaline is released from the adrenal, noradrenaline may be released from the postganglionic sympathetic nerve endings in the heart.[23]

The significance of sympathetic overactivity in relation to infarct size and ventricular dysrhythmias requires consideration. Sinus tachycardia was present in 24 per cent of patients seen within thirty minutes and appeared following the correction of vagal overactivity in a further 8 per cent. The adverse effect of sinus tachycardia on the ischaemic area surrounding the experimental infarct has been documented.[24, 25]

Ventricular Fibrillation Threshold

Stimulation of the cardiac sympathetic nerves gives rise to increased temporal dispersion of recovery and a fall in ventricular fibrillation threshold.[26, 27] Sympathetic denervation and beta-adrenoceptor-blocking agents will suppress the ventricular dysrhythmias produced by experimental coronary occlusion.[28, 29] Increase in the heart rate in the presence of ischaemia has been shown to cause a fall in the ventricular fibrillation threshold[30] and aggravates ventricular dysrhythmias.[31] In the clinical situation ventricular fibrillation may appear following the spontaneous increase in heart rate (Figure 12).

In summary, acute myocardial ischaemia leads to a fall in the ventricular fibrillation threshold. Autonomic imbalance causes a reduction in the ventricular fibrillation threshold. The high incidence of autonomic imbalance at the onset of acute myocardial infarction leads to a high risk of ventricular fibrillation (Table 3). It is clear, therefore, that in the management of the acute phase of myocardial infarction attention should be directed to the correction of both sympathetic and parasympathetic overactivity.

Importance of Early Intensive Care

It was postulated by Pantridge in 1970[12] that the early initiation of intensive care and the correction and prevention of dysrhythmias and autonomic disturbances might favourably influence the magnitude of the area of infarction (Figure 13). It has been stated

> . . .because myocardial tissue lies within the distribution of a recently occluded coronary artery does not mean that it is necessarily condemned to death. It is highly likely that the quantity of jeopardised myocardium that can be salvaged varies inversely with

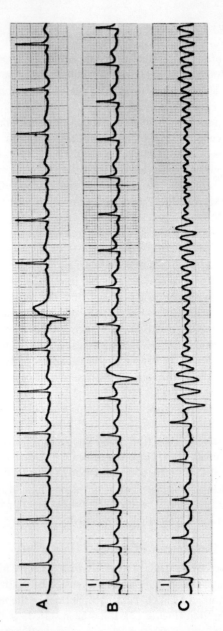

Figure 12 Lead 1, anterior infarct, estimated 55 minutes after onset of chest pain.
  A. Sinus rhythm (rate 95). Occasional 'benign' ventricular ectopics.
  B. Four minutes later, sinus tachycardia (rate 110) with ST segment elevation
     1.0 mm with one R on T ectopic.
  C. One minute after B, development of ventricular fibrillation before
     treatment could be given.

Table 3

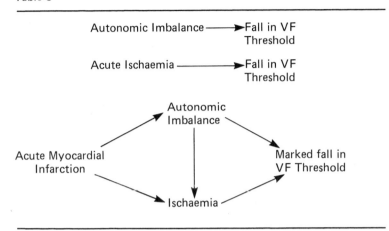

the time after coronary occlusion that the treatment is initiated.[32]

A low incidence of shock, pump failure and hospital fatality has been recorded among those seen early (Table 4). The hospital fatality of less than 10 per cent is to be contrasted with a fatality of 25.6 per cent among those patients in the Bristol study who contacted their doctors within one hour although they presumably did not have therapy within that time.[33] The difference in the relation to incidence of shock and pump failure between patients who came under intensive care within three hours and those who came under intensive care later is also shown in the Belfast data (Table 5).

Management of the Acute Phase of Myocardial Infarction

It is important to advise the patient to lie down immediately and request anyone who is near to seek urgent medical help. Immediate pain relief is regarded as particularly important in the management of acute myocardial infarction. Ectopic activity may subside when pain is relieved (Figure 14). The autonomic disturbances so frequent at the onset may respond to pain relief alone (Figure 15). The catechol release may be diminished by the immediate control of pain. Morphia is the drug most frequently administered. However, adverse effects have been documented. Profound hypotension and bradycardia may follow the administration of morphia, particularly when the patient is moved. Adverse haemodynamic effects also occur following the administration

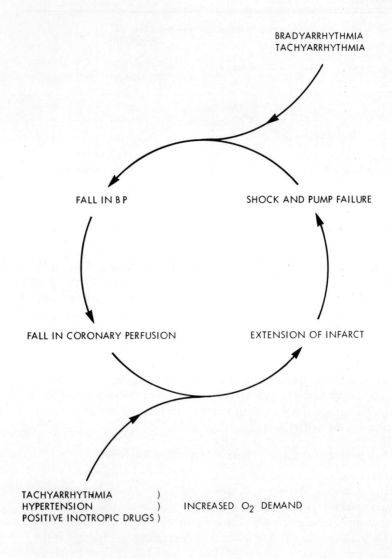

BRADYARRHYTHMIA
TACHYARRHYTHMIA

FALL IN B P

SHOCK AND PUMP FAILURE

FALL IN CORONARY PERFUSION

EXTENSION OF INFARCT

TACHYARRHYTHMIA   )
HYPERTENSION   )   INCREASED O₂ DEMAND
POSITIVE INOTROPIC DRUGS)

Figure 13 Uncorrected bradyarrhythmia and tachyarrhythmia in acute
    myocardial infarction

Table 4

	Patients Under 70 Years	Shock	Fatality
Prospective Study (1970-1973) (Pantridge et al., 1974)	271	9 (3.3%)	27 (< 10%)
Bristol Study (1971) (Mather et al., 1971)	117	Not recorded	30 (25.6%)

Table 5: Data on Patients Managed in 1969 by a Mobile Coronary Care Unit

Initiation of Coronary Care	Within 3 hours	After 3 hours
No. of Patients	319	128
Cardiogenic Shock*	14 (4%) (a)	17 (13%) (b)
Hospital Deaths**	31 (10%) (a)	24 (19%) (b)

*   (a) differs significantly from (b) $p = < 0.001$

** (a) differs significantly from (b) $0.01 > p > 0.001$

of pethidine to patients with acute myocardial infarction. Heroin is the most satisfactory of the narcotic drugs in the control of pain, particularly severe pain. Given in a standard intravenous dose of 5 mg, it causes little effect on the cardiovascular system. Usually the earlier the patient is seen the more severe the pain and higher doses of heroin are required. Heroin has a more rapid action and less emetic effect than morphia. Nevertheless, nausea and vomiting are relatively common in patients with acute myocardial infarction. Since vomiting causes adverse circulatory effects, it is important that it be controlled quickly. Heroin is, therefore, given in combination with an antiemetic. Cyclizine has been used but this drug has been found to increase the heart rate which is undesirable in patients with a normal or already increased heart rate. Metoclopramide monohydrochloride (Maxolon) is a suitable alternative to cyclizine.

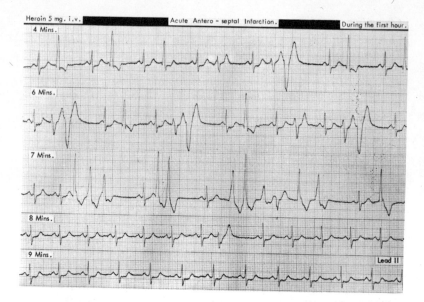

Figure 14 Record at an estimated 50 minutes after the onset of acute anterior infarction during severe chest pain. Heart rate 90/minute with frequent salvos of ventricular ectopics; blood pressure 170/100 mm Hg. Nine minutes after the administration of diamorphine 5 mg intravenously, heart rate 80/minute with disappearance of ventricular dysrhythmias; blood pressure 160/90 mm Hg. No antiarrhythmic therapy was given.

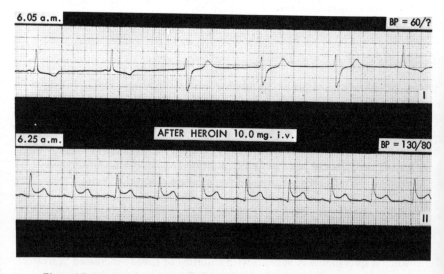

Figure 15 Record at an estimated 60 minutes after the onset of acute diaphragmatic infarction. Sinus bradycardia 45/minute with idioventricular rhythm. Blood pressure 60/ ? mm. After heroin 10 mg intravenously sinus rhythm 83/minute, blood pressure 130/80.

Correction of Autonomic Disturbance

Sinus bradycardia does not require therapy unless it is accompanied by hypotension or ventricular ectopics. However, uncomplicated bradyarrhythmia in the acute phase of myocardial infarction is uncommon. The correction of bradyarrhythmia may be achieved by increasing the heart rate by the administration of atropine. The importance of correcting hypotension is indicated by the mortality of hypotensive patients in the Bristol study. Patients in that study who had a systolic blood pressure less than 100 mm mercury had a fatality of 49 per cent.[33] However, of the 294 patients seen and managed by the mobile coronary care unit within one hour hypotensive patients had a mortality of 16 per cent. Bradycardia accompanied the hypotension in 71 per cent.[34]

When atropine is required for the correction of sinus bradycardia it is administered in aliquots of 0.3 to 0.6 mg intravenously (Figure 16). The electrocardiogram is continuously monitored at the time of administration. Increase in the heart rate is usually accompanied by an increase in the blood pressure. Indeed, 28 (80 per cent) of 35 patients with the bradycardia-hypotension syndrome seen within one hour of the onset of infarction showed a rise in blood pressure following the administration of atropine. Atropine is often indicated in nodal bradycardia since the loss of atrial transport function usually accentuates hypotension. Early complete atrio-ventricular block frequently responds to atropine (Figure 17).

It is known that relatively little vagal overactivity usually overpowers even marked sympathetic overactivity.[35] Thus, atropine is administered in small aliquots under monitoring control since reduction of vagal overactivity may unmask sympathetic overactivity and lead to an inappropriately rapid heart rate (Figure 17). Sudden unmasking of sympathetic overactivity may precipitate ventricular fibrillation (Figure 18). Despite careful titration of the dosage, atropine gave rise to sinus tachycardia in over one fifth of the patients with bradycardia and hypotension.

Practolol, a selective cardiac beta-adrenergic-blocking agent in a dose of 10 mg intravenously or sotalol in a similar dosage is effective in the control of sinus tachycardia (Figure 19). Sotalol, which does not possess intrinsic sympathomimetic activity, appears to have a more potent negative chronotropic effect than practolol.

Practolol was effective in the control of sympathetic overactivity unmasked by atropine (Figure 20). Reduction in ST segment elevation

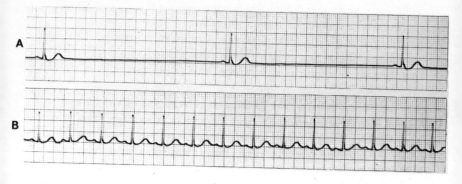

Figure 16 Record at an estimated 50 minutes after the onset of acute posterior infarction.
    A. Sinus bradycardia 16/minute, blood pressure 60/?
    B. After atropine 0.9 mg intravenously sinus rhythm 100/minute, blood pressure 120/90.

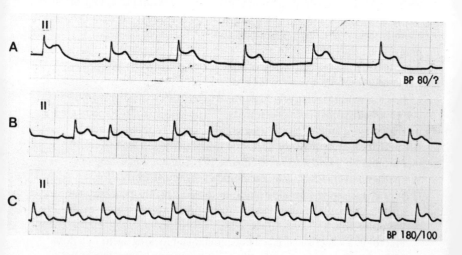

Figure 17 Record at an estimated 45 minutes after the onset of acute posterior infarction.
    A. Atrial rate 70; ventricular rate 56; systolic blood pressure 80 mm Hg.
    B. Three minutes after atropine 2.8 mg intravenously. Second degree atrioventricular block (Wenckebach).
    C. Five minutes after atropine 2.8 mg intravenously. Sinus tachycardia and transient hypertension. Normal atrio-ventricular conduction.

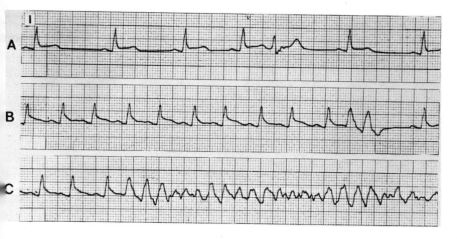

Figure 18 Anterior infarction lead 1.
- A. Sinus bradycardia (rate 55) with ventricular ectopic.
- B. Two minutes after atropine 0.6 mg intravenously, sinus tachycardia (rate 110) with consecutive ventricular ectopics.
- C. Three minutes after atropine, development of ventricular fibrillation.

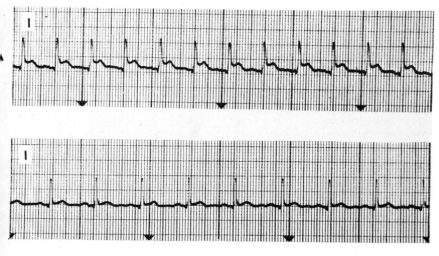

Figure 19 Effect of sotalol on sinus tachycardia in a normotensive patient with anterior infarction. Lead 1 recorded an estimated 40 minutes after onset of infarction.
- A. Sinus tachycardia (rate 125). ST segment elevation 2.5 mm.
- B. Six minutes after sotalol 10 mg intravenously: rate 96, ST elevation 0.5 mm, no significant reduction in blood pressure.

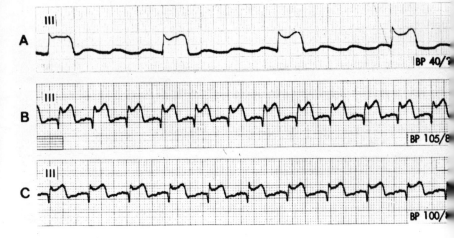

Figure 20 Effect of practolol on sympathetic overactivity unmasked by atropine.
- A. Acute posterior infarction, complete heart block; ventricular rate 33/minute, systolic blood pressure 40 mm Hg.
- B. Sinus tachycardia (rate 112/minute) following atropine 2.4 mg intravenously; ST segment elevation 3.0 mm.
- C. Ten minutes after practolol 5 mg intravenously; sinus rhythm (rate 96/minute), ST segment elevation 1.5 mm.

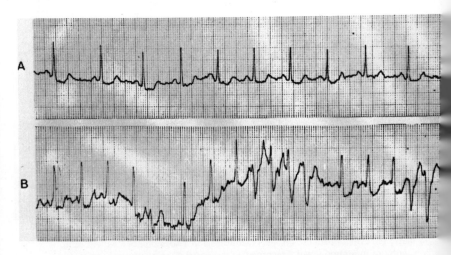

Figure 21 Records obtained within one hour of the onset of acute anterior infarction.
- A. Before movement to the ambulance. Heart rate 90/minute, blood pressure 160/90 mm Hg. No ventricular ectopics.
- B. During movement to the ambulance. Heart rate 130/minute with salvos of ventricular ectopics.

accompanied the fall in heart rate. The decrease in ST segment elevation is likely to indicate a reduction in the ischaemic injury surrounding the infarct.

Autonomic disturbance and ventricular dysrhythmias are often exacerbated or appear for the first time during movement of patients with acute myocardial infarction (Figure 21). Thus, a heart rate of 110/minute or greater occurred during transport in over one third of patients.[36] These patients were transported to a community hospital in ordinary ambulances, the drivers of which had been supplied with simple monitoring equipment. Pain relief prior to transport had no effect on the incidence of a rapid heart rate. The prophylactic administration of practolol proved to be of limited value but sotalol usually prevented the heart rate exceeding 110/minute.

Ventricular Ectopics

It is usually considered that frequent, multifocal or R on T ventricular ectopics occurring in patients in coronary care units are associated with a high risk of ventricular fibrillation and constitute an indication for immediate antiarrhythmic therapy. The value of lignocaine in the control of ventricular ectopics in the coronary care unit is well documented. However, in 1970, data were presented suggesting that lignocaine in standard dosage was of limited value in the control of ventricular dysrhythmias occurring within one hour of the onset of infarction.[37] Lignocaine abolished ventricular ectopic activity completely in only 27 per cent of patients and in 38 per cent it had no effect. Subsequent studies showed that lignocaine may be without effect even in the presence of relatively high blood levels of the drug.

The high incidence of autonomic disturbance in the very early phase of acute myocardial infarction may explain the limited response to lignocaine observed at that time. The effect of lignocaine in suppressing ventricular ectopics may be rate related. It proved less effective in the presence of sinus tachycardia (Figures 22 and 23). When the heart rate was between 60 and 90/minute (Figure 23) the drug had a beneficial effect on ectopic activity in 70 per cent of patients and had no effect or increased the ventricular dysrhythmia in 30 per cent. However, when the rate was over 90/minute ectopic activity was diminished or abolished in only 36 per cent and was unaffected or increased in 64 per cent. An increase in ventricular ectopic activity following the intravenous administration of lignocaine in the presence of sinus tachycardia has been reported by others. Ectopic activity in patients with heart rates above 90/minute who are not in heart failure is now

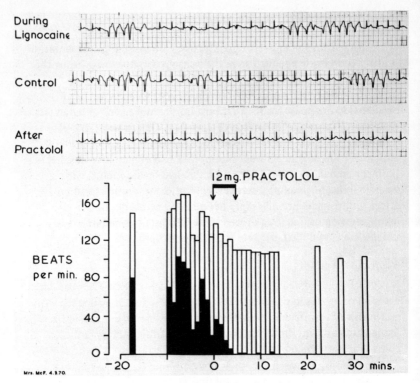

Figure 22 Black columns — ventricular ectopics. Clear columns — heart rate. Effect of practolol on lignocaine-resistant multiform ventricular ectopics and ventricular tachycardia four hours after resuscitation from ventricular fibrillation.

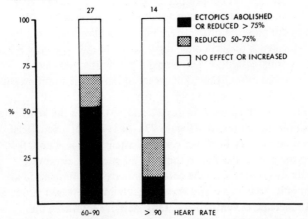

Figure 23 The effect of lignocaine 100 mg intravenously followed by 2 mg/minute on ventricular ectopic activity in 41 patients treated within four hours of the onset of symptoms. The heart rate was between 60 and 90/minute in 27 patients and over 90/minute in 14.

managed by reducing the rate with a beta-blocking agent. Lignocaine might then be administered if required. When the heart rate is greater than 90/minute, practolol or sotalol gives a significant reduction in rate.

Ventricular Tachycardia

Ventricular tachycardia appearing soon after the onset of symptoms is frequently accompanied by marked hypotension. The administration of lignocaine in this situation may be hazardous. Ventricular tachycardia may be terminated by a sharp precordial blow. When a patient with ventricular tachycardia complicated by profound hypotension is seen outside hospital a direct current shock, even if unsynchronised, is likely to be safer than lignocaine.

Ventricular Fibrillation

Very occasionally ventricular fibrillation may be self-terminating (Figure 24). Occasionally ventricular fibrillation may be corrected by a chest blow (Figure 25). However, direct current defibrillation is almost always required.

It is now well established that medical and paramedical personnel are capable of correcting ventricular fibrillation outside hospital. Cobb's paramedical scheme in Seattle has been particularly successful.[38] Among the patients resuscitated from ventricular fibrillation during the third year of the unit's operation there were sixty-four long-term survivors and during the fourth year seventy-three long-term survivors (Figure 26).

The widespread availability of defibrillators is clearly desirable and, indeed, Friedberg[39] has indicated that those at risk should have a defibrillator at hand, even when at home. A major barrier to the general availability of defibrillators for use outside hospital by general practitioners, paramedical individuals and others relates to the fact that it is widely assumed that the energy required for defibrillation is high. It is generally taught that 'the highest energy setting should always be used'.[40] Some of the portable defibrillators available at present are cumbersome, heavy and expensive. Some weigh as much as 55 lb (25 kg). Furthermore, it has been said by Tacker and his colleagues[41] that the energy delivered from defibrillators at present available may be insufficient to achieve defibrillation in large individuals. They claim that the energy delivered by most commercially available defibrillators, 300 Joules, from a stored energy of 400, is unlikely to be effective in 50 per cent of patients weighing 82 kg and have shown it to be ineffective in 60 per cent of patients weighing between 90 and 100 kg.

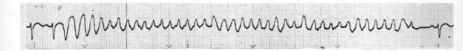

Figure 24   Self-terminating ventricular fibrillation

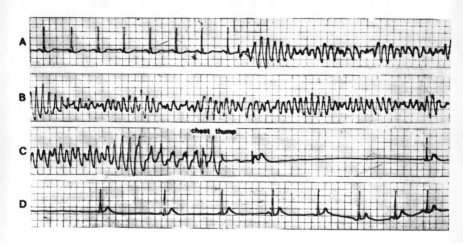

Figure 25   Primary ventricular fibrillation in a 55-year-old man with acute
posterior infarction.
   A. Sinus rhythm (heart rate 75/minute, blood pressure 130/90 mm Hg).
      Development of primary ventricular fibrillation without warning
      dysrhythmias.
   B. Continuous with A.
   C. Chest thump followed by asystole and atrio-ventricular junctional
      escape rhythm.
   D. Continuous with C. Restoration of sinus rhythm.

SEATTLE

Ventricular Fibrillation
present on arrival

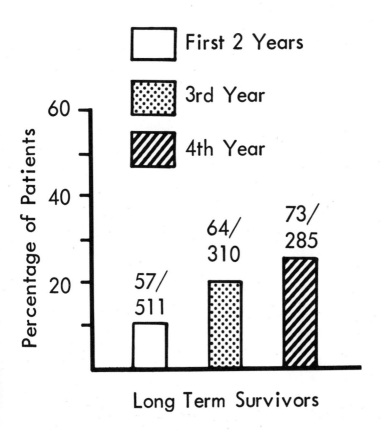

Figure 26 Seattle: patients with ventricular fibrillation on arrival

This implies that the trend should be towards the production of larger defibrillators. Their findings, however, are not in accordance with the experience of others. A shock of 300 Joules successfully defibrillated a patient weighing 145 kg.[42] It has been observed that shocks of 150-165 Joules were effective in removing ventricular fibrillation.[43]

In the belief that the trend should be towards smaller, cheaper and therefore more readily available defibrillators, a miniature instrument (Pantridge defibrillator) was designed, weighing less than 7 lb (3.2 kg) (Figures 27 and 28). The electronic components are incorporated in the paddles. From a stored energy of 400 Joules, 330 are delivered through a resistance of 50 ohms and 165 Joules are delivered from a stored energy of 200. The battery is capable of delivering 25 direct current shocks of 400 Joules before recharge.

In Belfast, the efficacy of low energy shocks was investigated in 233 episodes of ventricular fibrillation in 120 patients, the majority of whom had had an acute myocardial infarction. Two types of defibrillators were used, each charged to 200 Joules. From this stored energy the American Optical apparatus delivered 150 Joules through a resistance of 50 ohms and the Pantridge defibrillator 165 Joules. When the initial shock failed to remove the ventricular fibrillation, a further identical low energy shock was applied immediately. In one patient, a single 100 Joules discharge was successful. The effect of each shock was observed on a continuous recording of the electrocardiogram on paper. The incidence of successful defibrillation related to body weight is shown in Figure 29. In 95 per cent of the episodes low energy shocks were successful. Eighty-five per cent were successfully defibrillated by a single 200 shock. In 9 per cent a second low energy shock was successful. In patients weighing more than 80 kg, 90 per cent of the episodes were successfully defibrillated by low energy shocks. The heaviest individual weighed 102 kg. Low energy defibrillation was successful in 95 per cent of 150 episodes of primary ventricular fibrillation and in 98 per cent that occurred within one hour of myocardial infarction.

Defibrillation with low energy shocks has merit apart from that related to the diminution in weight and size of the defibrillators. The lower the energy of the shock the less the myocardial damage. In buildings occupied by a large number of individuals, particularly middle-aged males, it might be appropriate to mount portable defibrillators beside the fire extinguishers (Figure 30). Furthermore, a portable defibrillator should be part of the equipment of general practitioners and physicians who are likely to be involved in medical

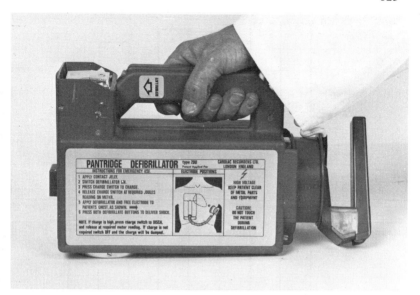

Figure 27 The miniature DC defibrillator

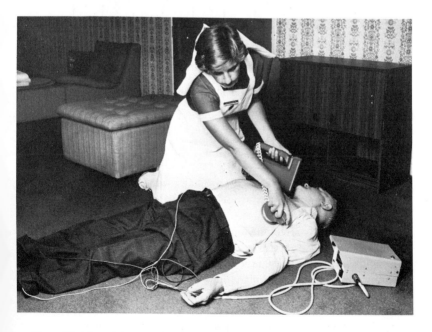

Figure 28 The miniature defibrillator in use

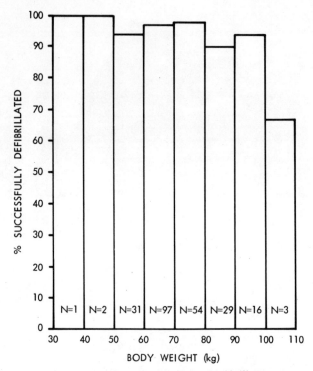

N = Number of episodes of ventricular fibrillation

Figure 29   Incidence of successful defibrillation with low energy shocks related to body weight

emergencies.

The long-term prognosis of survivors following ventricular fibrillation is similar to that of patients whose myocardial infarction is not so complicated.[44, 45] The number of episodes of ventricular fibrillation does not adversely affect the long-term prognosis. Patients who survive ventricular fibrillation that occurs within four hours of the onset of symptoms are younger, tend to have had a mild coronary attack, and have the most favourable long-term prognosis (Figure 31).[45]

Conclusions

There is at present no procrustean approach to the correction of dysrhythmias and the autonomic disturbance so frequently present in

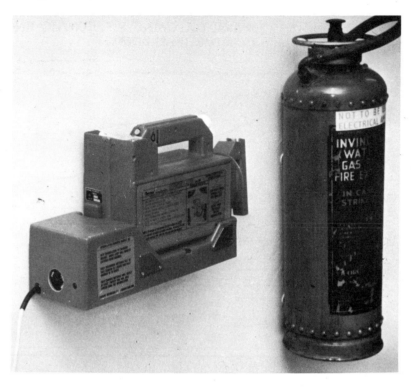

Figure 30 Miniature defibrillator sitting in its charging unit and mounted beside the fire extinguisher

the acute phase of myocardial infarction. Careful titration of the dose of the necessary drugs is required. Since the dysrhythmias and the autonomic disturbance influence the magnitude of the infarct and, therefore, the incidence of shock, pump failure, and long-term prognosis, there will continue to be a place for the operation of mobile coronary care units staffed by physicians or general practitioners. All that is required is an individual trained in coronary care with the necessary equipment and means of transport. The latter might, indeed, be the general practitioner's or junior doctor's car. The development of a simplified therapeutic regime for the stabilisation of the rhythm, the autonomic difficulty and the haemodynamic state is essential. If such a regime evolves, it might be initiated not only by medical or para-medical personnel but also in some situations by the patient

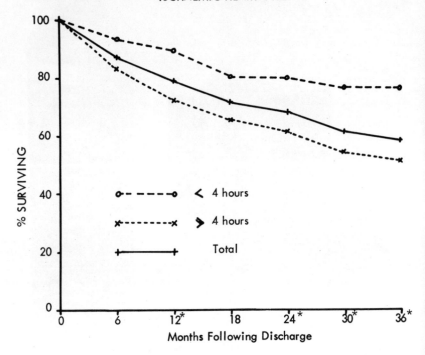

Figure 31 Survival of patients who had ventricular fibrillation less than four hours after the onset of symptoms of acute myocardial ischaemia compared with that of patients who had ventricular fibrillation later

* $P < 0.05$.

himself. Highly efficient automatic spring injectors exist. The drugs to be carried in such syringes and the dosage are problems to be solved.

Notes

1. Bainton, C.R. and Peterson, D.R., 'Deaths from Coronary Heart Disease in Persons Fifty Years of Age and Younger', *New England Journal of Medicine*, 1963, 268, 569.
2. Gordon, T. and Kannel, W.B., 'Premature Mortality from Coronary Heart

Disease: The Framingham Study', *Journal of the American Medical Association,* 1971, 215, 1617.
3. Adgey, A.A.J. *et al.,* 'Management of Ventricular Fibrillation outside Hospital', *Lancet,* 1969, 1, 1169.
4. Pantridge, J.F. and Adgey, A.A.J., 'Pre-Hospital Coronary Care: The Mobile Coronary Care Unit', *American Journal of Cardiology,* 1969, 24, 666.
5. Von Bezold, A. and Hirt, L., 'Ueber Die Physiologischen Wirkungen des Essigsauren Veratrins', *Untersuch. Physiol. Lab. Wurzburg,* 1867, 1, 75.
6. Juhasz-Nagy, A. and Szentivanyi, M., 'Localisation of the Receptors of the Coronary Chemoreflex in the Dog', *Archives Internationales de Pharmacodynamie et de Thérapie,* 1961, 131, 39.
7. Frink, R.J. and James, T.N., 'Intracardiac Route of the Bezold-Jarisch Reflex', *American Journal of Physiology,* 1971, 221, 1464.
8. Adgey, A.A.J. *et al.,* 'Incidence, Significance, and Management of Early Brady-arrhythmia Complicating Acute Myocardial Infarction', *Lancet,* 1968, 2, 1097.
9. Sarnoff, S.J. *et al.,* 'Regulation of Ventricular Contraction: Influence of Cardiac Sympathetic and Vagal Nerve Stimulation on Atrial and Ventricular Dynamics', *Circulation Research,* 1960, 8, 1108.
10. DeGeest, H. *et al.,* 'Depression of Ventricular Contractility by Stimulation of the Vagus Nerves', *Circulation Research,* 1965, 17, 222.
11. Wildenthal, K. *et al.,* 'Influence of Efferent Vagal Stimulation on Left Ventricular Function in Dogs', *American Journal of Physiology,* 1969, 216, 577.
12. Pantridge, J.F., 'The Effect of Early Therapy on the Hospital Mortality from Acute Myocardial Infarction', *Quarterly Journal of Medicine,* 1970, 39, 621.
13. Lawrie, D.M. *et al.,* 'A Coronary Care Unit in the Routine Management of Acute Myocardial Infarction', *Lancet,* 1967, 2, 109.
14. George, M. and Greenwood, T.W., 'Relation between Bradycardia and the Site of Myocardial Infarction', *Lancet,* 1967, 2, 739.
15. Norris, R.M., 'Bradyarrhythmia after Myocardial Infarction', *Lancet,* 1969, 1, 313.
16. Cannom, D.S., Harrison, D.C. and Schroeder, J.S., 'Hemodynamic Observations in Patients with Unstable Angina Pectoris', *American Journal of Cardiology,* 1974, 33, 17.
17. Gazes, P.C., Richardson, J.A. and Woods E.F., 'Plasma Catecholamine Concentrations in Myocardial Infarction and Angina Pectoris', *Circulation,* 1959, 19, 657.
18. McDonald, L. *et al.,* 'Plasma-catecholamines after Cardiac Infarction', *Lancet,* 1969, 2, 1021.
19. Nelson, P.G., 'Effect of Heparin on Serum Free Fatty Acids, Plasma Catecholamines and the Incidence of Arrhythmias Following Acute Myocardial Infarction', *British Medical Journal,* 1970, 3, 735.
20. Vetter, N.J. *et al.,* 'Initial Metabolic and Hormonal Response to Acute Myocardial Infarction', *Lancet,* 1974, 1, 284.
21. Brown, A.M., 'Excitation of Afferent Cardiac Sympathetic Nerve Fibres During Myocardial Ischaemia', *Journal of Physiology,* 1967, 190, 35.
22. Malliani, A., Schwartz, P.J. and Zanchetti, A., 'A Sympathetic Reflex Elicited by Experimental Coronary Occlusion', *American Journal of Physiology,* 1969, 217, 703.
23. Staszewska-Barczak, J., 'The Reflex Stimulation of Catecholamine Secretion During the Acute Stage of Myocardial Infarction in the Dog', *Clinical Science,* 1971, 41, 419.
24. Maroko, P.R. *et al.,* 'Factors Influencing Infarct Size Following Experimental

Coronary Artery Occlusions', *Circulation,* 1971, 43, 67.

25. Shell, W.E. and Sobel, B.E., 'Deleterious Effects of Increased Heart Rate on Infarct Size in the Conscious Dog', *American Journal of Cardiology,* 1973, 31, 474.

26. Han, J. and Moe, G.K., 'Non-uniform Recovery of Excitability of Ventricular Muscle', *Circulation Research,* 1964, 14, 44.

27. Han, J., DeJalon, P.G. and Moe, G.K., 'Adrenergic Effects on Ventricular Vulnerability', *Circulation Research,* 1964, 14, 516.

28. Ebert, P.A., Allgood, R.J. and Sabiston, D.C. Jr., 'Effect of Cardiac Denervation on Arrhythmia Following Coronary Artery Occlusion', *Surgical Forum,* 1967, 18, 114.

29. Ceremuzynski, L., Staszewska-Barczak, J. and Herbaczynska-Cedro, K., 'Cardiac Rhythm Disturbances and the Release of Catecholamines after Acute Coronary Occlusion in Dogs', *Cardiovascular Research,* 1969, 3, 190.

30. Kent, K.M. *et al.,* 'Electrical Stability of Acutely Ischaemic Myocardium: Influences of Heart Rate and Vagal Stimulation', *Circulation,* 1973, 47, 291.

31. Scherlag, B.J. *et al.,* Electrophysiology Underlying Ventricular Arrhythmias Due to Coronary Ligation', *American Journal of Physiology,* 1970, 219, 1665.

32. Braunwald, E., 'Reduction of Myocardial Infarct Size', *New England Journal of Medicine,* 1974, 291, 526.

33. Mather, H.G. *et al.,* 'Acute Myocardial Infarction: Home and Hospital Treatment', *British Medical Journal,* 1971, 4, 334.

34. Pantridge, J.F. *et al.,* 'The First Hour after the Onset of Acute Myocardial Infarction', in *Progress in Cardiology,* vol.III (edited by Yu, P.N. and Goodwin, J.F.), p.173. Philadelphia, Lea and Febiger.

35. Samaan, A., 'The Antagonistic Cardiac Nerves and Heart Rate', *Journal of Physiology,* 1935, 83, 332.

36. Mulholland, H.C. and Pantridge, J.F., 'Heart Rate Changes During Movement of Patients with Acute Myocardial Infarction', *Lancet,* 1974, 1, 1244.

37. Pantridge, J.F., 'Emergency Treatment of Cardiac Arrhythmias in Myocardial Infarction', in *Lidocaine in the Treatment of Ventricular Arrhythmias: Proceedings of a Symposium* (edited by Scott, D.B. and Julian, D.G.), p.77. Edinburgh, E. and S. Livingstone.

38. Cobb, L.A. *et al.,* 'Resuscitation from Out-of-Hospital Ventricular Fibrillation, Four Years Follow Up', *Circulation,* 1975, 51 and 52, Supplement III, 223-8.

39. Friedberg, C.K., 'Introduction: Symposium, Myocardial Infarction (Part 1)', *Circulation,* 1972, 45, 179.

40. Dunning, A.J., 'The Treatment of Ventricular Fibrillation', in *Textbook of Coronary Care* (edited by Meltzer, L.E. and Dunning, A.J.), p.371. Amsterdam, Excerpta Medica.

41. Tacker, W.A. Jr. *et al.,* 'Energy Dose for Human Trans-Chest Electrical Ventricular Defibrillation', *New England Journal of Medicine,* 1974, 290, 214.

42. Lappin, H.A., 'Ventricular Defibrillators in Heavy Patients', *New England Journal of Medicine,* 1974, 291, 153.

43. Pantridge, J.F. *et al.,* 'Electrical Requirements for Ventricular Defibrillation', *British Medical Journal,* 1975, 2, 313.

44. Geddes, J.S., Adgey, A.A.J. and Pantridge, J.F., 'Prognosis after Recovery from Ventricular Fibrillation Complicating Ischaemic Heart Disease', *Lancet,* 1967, 2, 273.

45. McNamee, B.T. *et al.,* 'Long-term Prognosis Following Ventricular Fibrillation in Acute Ischaemic Heart Disease', *British Medical Journal,* 1970, 4, 204.

46. McNeilly, R.H. and Pemberton, J., 'Duration of Last Attack in 998 Fatal Cases of Coronary Artery Disease and Its Relation to Possible Cardiac

Resuscitation', *British Medical Journal,* 1968, 3, 139.
47. Armstrong, A. *et al.,* 'Natural History of Acute Coronary Heart Attacks: A Community Study', *British Heart Journal,* 1972, 34, 67.

8 THE USE OF AMBULANCEMEN IN PRE-HOSPITAL CORONARY CARE

Dr Douglas Chamberlain

History of the Scheme

Following the impressive results achieved by Professor Pantridge and his colleagues in Belfast,[1] a coronary ambulance system was instituted in the County Borough of Brighton in 1969 by Dr William Parker who was then Medical Officer of Health. Unfortunately, as far as Brighton was concerned, this was ahead of its time. There was no coronary care unit, there was no medical or nursing staff available to man the ambulance and the scheme did not prosper. When attempts to use hospital staff proved impracticable Dr Parker tried to launch a scheme run by general practitioners, but this too did not work. In twelve months, up to 1970, the ambulance had been called out only eight times.

I arrived in Brighton in June 1970 and at first was only vaguely aware of the existence of the ambulance. I had no wish to become involved with it, partly because I believed that pre-hospital coronary care could never be cost-effective. My first encounter with the ambulance — and with Dr Parker — occurred towards the end of 1970 when a patient I was visiting at home developed ventricular fibrillation. Due to a series of misunderstandings it took a long time for the ambulance to arrive and when it did so a component of the defibrillator exploded. It was under these inauspicious circumstances that Dr Parker and I decided that we should work together to make the system effective. We agreed that the best prospect lay in training the ambulancemen to carry out the necessary procedures themselves without immediate aid or supervision. We believed we were pioneering a new method, unaware of the experience already being gained with coronary ambulances staffed by paramedical personnel in the United States,[2] and, on a smaller scale, in Dublin.[3]

The scheme we operate now is basically the same as the one we planned in 1970.[4, 5] It has not yet reached its full potential for reasons which I shall mention, and some of our ideas about equipment have of course changed over the last five years. Our view on what skilled attendants can achieve and how they should be trained are unchanged. We believe that the ambulancemen who are responsible for resuscitations should understand very clearly everything that they see in patients they are caring for. A very comprehensive training in coronary artery disease therefore seems important. The object has always been for a level of skill which will enable ambulancemen to give selected drugs intravenously or intramuscularly, to intubate patients and to set up infusions. This in fact is the way things are developing. From the very beginning, then, our concept has been not so much of coronary ambulances as of resuscitation ambulances.

Training Ambulancemen in Coronary Care

The initial training of the ambulancemen comprises twenty-four lectures of 1½ hours each, given jointly to themselves and to the nurses on our coronary care course. Approximately half of that period of ninety minutes is spent on revision, in the form of questions, to the participants; the subsequent forty-five minutes are spent teaching something new. The lectures cover some anatomy and physiology of the circulation, the pathology and clinical presentation of coronary disease, and the problems which follow from its major complications; we teach electrocardiography to a relatively high standard, particularly the dysrhythmias; and we deal with the pharmacology of all the commonly used cardio-active drugs. The ambulancemen also spend one month full-time in the coronary care unit, so that they gain experience in putting on electrodes, taking electrocardiograms, coping with any 'cold' defibrillations and helping generally to care for patients. At the end of this course they have a stiff examination consisting of a written paper, the identification of twenty dysrhythmias, a practical test on resuscitation procedures, and a general viva. Although the pass standard is high (requiring 70 per cent of possible marks), most are successful and are declared proficient to defibrillate patients. Those who fail can take the examination again six months later if they choose. Subsequently, having had about six months experience on the ambulance, they return for a second examination; if they prove themselves particularly skilled in the interpretation of dysrhythmias and in the basic clinical pharmacology of lignocaine and atropine, we permit them to give these drugs intravenously in carefully defined circumstances. As a third stage they are trained by some of our anaesthetists in intubation techniques. The purpose of the intubation training is to enable ambulancemen to deal more effectively with cases of drowning, drug overdose and perhaps major injury. In the event it has proved of greater value than we expected in the management of cardiac emergencies. Finally, we teach them about infusion techniques, again with a view to treating traumatic shock.

By early 1974 we had reached the stage of having some 28 men trained to defibrillate, 19 for drug administration, 7 for intubation and 2 for infusion techniques.

At that stage the reorganisation of the Health Service occurred, and as far as we were concerned this was initially a near disaster. We lost Dr Parker, who had initiated the scheme and been a tremendous help with its development. He is still a community physician but no longer involved directly with the ambulances. We also lost our ambulance chief who had given invaluable assistance in developing the system. For many months nobody was in a position to authorise further training and morale suffered considerably. When eventually an Area Chief Ambulance Officer was appointed he was unconvinced of the merits of resuscitation ambulances just as I had been earlier. A further set-back occurred when a new national salary agreement revoked the 10 per cent special salary allowance which the extra training had attracted, and indeed three months supplementary pay was to be reclaimed!

Fortunately the crises have now passed. The Area Chief Ambulance Officer has made his own major contribution to the organisation of the system which now comprises three ambulances, two stationed in Brighton and one in Hove. This distribution permits a median response time (call received to arrival with patient) of only five minutes. All the stretcher-carrying ambulances can quickly be fitted with the portable resuscitation equipment, so no vehicles need to be designated permanently for this function. The increased flexibility has important operational advantages. Although the special skills of the trained attendants no longer attracts 10 per cent of their new salary, the weekly supplement paid in 1974 has been restored (but as salaries increase, this of course becomes an ever-decreasing benefit in percentage terms). Finally, permission has recently been given for a limited resumption of training. This is of prime importance because eight of those previously trained have now been upgraded to control duties and no longer undertake routine work on the ambulances.

Calling the Ambulance

How is a resuscitation ambulance summoned? If a doctor requesting the transfer of a patient gives a diagnosis which suggests a myocardial infarction or 'coronary' then the special ambulance will be sent, unless the doctor specifies otherwise, which would be unlikely. Moreover, we encourage doctors *not* to visit patients first after receiving emergency calls for chest pains or collapse; ideally both doctor and ambulance should set out together, and this system often works well. The doctor may not be able to attend quickly but the ambulance can; the patient then is usually taken directly to hospital, but the attendants may use their discretion and report back to the general practitioner. Moreover, a resuscitation ambulance will be used in response to any emergency call from any source if there is a suggestion of collapse, unconsciousness, serious chest pain or major injury. Calls made by or on behalf of patients with previous coronary disease also receive special consideration.

During the two years 1974 and 1975, 2,253 calls were considered by ambulance control as requiring the special vehicles. Retrospective diagnoses of the patients carried showed that 30 per cent had acute myocardial infarction and 20 per cent had coronary insufficiency or some other cardiac problem. Fifty per cent of calls were for conditions not requiring cardiac or resuscitation facilities and included patients who were found dead when a cardiac cause could not be established. It also included a wide variety of other conditions such as non-cardiac chest pain, fractures, epilepsy, as well as a small number of apparently spurious calls. In other words, resuscitation ambulances were used appropriately in about half the cases, but most of the other calls also required a stretcher-bearing ambulance so that few journeys were 'wasted'. It must be stressed that designated vehicles were also used for non-urgent duties when pressure of work demanded. Such journeys have not been included in the total. The use of special ambulances reduces delay in the admission of coronary patients to hospital. Of all the patients admitted to the coronary care unit in 1974 and 1975, 3 per cent were admitted in less than half an hour, 17 per cent in less than an hour and 41 per cent in less than two hours from the onset of the attack. But for those patients who travelled in the special ambulances, the figures were 6 per cent, 30 per cent and 54 per cent respectively. These figures do not include the cases for which we had inadequate data, usually because the onset of major symptoms could not be defined accurately. There was a marked difference in the response time between '999' calls and general practitioner calls. The median times for the ambulance to reach the patients were respectively 24 minutes and 131 minutes for these two groups. This difference is not the fault of general practitioners, for the cases were different. For example, if a patient collapses in the street a '999' call is usually made very quickly whereas a patient developing chest pain at home seeks help much more slowly.

When the ambulance reaches its destination, the portable defibrillator/oscilloscope unit (Simonsen and Weel, DMS 200) is taken to the patient. Inside the lid of the unit there is a tape recorder (National Panasonic RQ 212 DF) which stores a modulated ECG signal for subsequent analysis within the coronary care unit. It is left switched on during all patient monitoring. A Siemens Cardiostat electrocardiograph is also attached and can provide a permanent record of any signal seen on the oscilloscope. Assuming that a very rapid assessment does not *exclude* a possible cardiac amergency, an initial single-lead electrocardiogram is taken before the patient is moved, to confirm and document that the heart rhythm is not obviously unstable. In an emergency, with a collapsed patient, the rhythm is recorded through defibrillation paddles (Figure 1) and if ventricular fibrillation is identified, an appropriate shock can be given without delay. Whether or not any immediate treatment is required, the patient's heart rhythm is monitored throughout the journey to hospital using the relatively large and clear memory display on the portable oscilloscope. This is mounted in the ambulance in such a way that the attendant can readily see the screen and the patient at the same time. On arrival at hospital the ambulance attendant hands in the tape cassette and a report sheet which includes a list of any abnormalities of heart rhythm which were observed.

Accuracy of ECG Diagnosis and Proficiency in the Use of Drugs

The tapes are all analysed by an experienced Senior House Officer, and usually there is complete agreement with the ambulanceman's diagnosis. Of 3,158 rhythms recorded in 2,180 patients in 1974 and 1975, there was agreement in 94 per cent. If tapes which showed only sinus rhythm are excluded, the agreement is still 90 per cent. Moreover, not all the remaining 10 per cent represented errors. For example, there were six instances of ventricular fibrillation reported by the ambulancemen not seen by the Senior House Officer. These discrepancies occurred because attendants omitted to turn on the tape recorders in the excitement of dealing with collapsed patients. This understandable but irritating omission is now prevented by automatic switching when the portable equipment is used in any way. Other disagreements — for example between sinus tachycardia and supraventricular tachycardia — could sometimes be explained by poor quality of signals in restless patients. The high level of competence in the recognition of dysrhythmias justified our decision to allow ambulancemen to give drugs in certain emergencies.

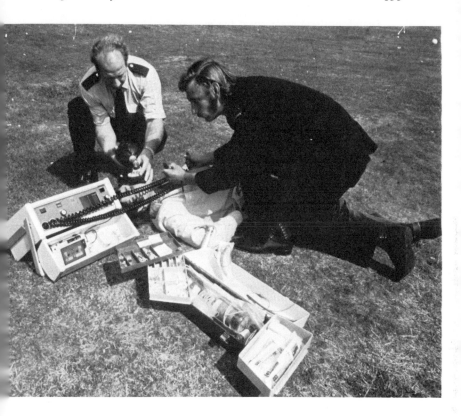

Figure 1 The use of a combined monitoring oscilloscope/defibrillator by an ambulanceman. Large insulated hand-held 'paddles' can be used as emergency chest electrodes to pick up the electrocardiogram which is displayed on a large screen. The same 'paddles' can deliver high energy shocks to the heart if ventricular fibrillation is diagnosed.

Only four drugs are given at the present time. These are: intravenous atropine for serious bradydysrhythmias or in the presence of ventricular irritability if the basic rate is abnormally slow (Figure 2); intravenous lignocaine for other ventricular tachydysrhythmias following conventional indications; Entonox (50 per cent nitrous oxide and 50 per cent oxygen) for patients with pain; and dexamethasone for patients who remain unconscious after resuscitation. We prefer this to be given in the ambulance because in the past there has sometimes been inadvertent serious delay in its administration in the hospital. The indications, doses and methods of administration of these drugs are very closely defined, and particular care is taken in checking these points retrospectively.

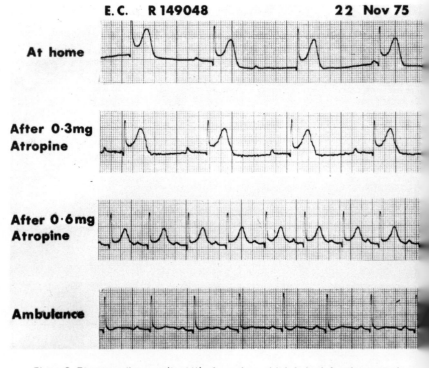

Figure 2 Electrocardiograms (lead II) of a patient with inferior infarction treated with intravenous atropine by an ambulanceman. The first tracing shows bradycardia (40 per minute), complete heart block and 4 mm ST elevation. Conduction with 2nd degree (2:1) block returned after 0.3 mg atropine. The dose was repeated and normal conduction at 75 beats per minute was achieved before the patient was moved. The ECG abnormality during the ambulance journey was relatively slight.

Table 1 summarises the results of the administration of atropine and lignocaine by the ambulancemen in 1974 and 1975. A total of 127 patients were given atropine, and in no case was the indication incorrect; for one patient, no tape or ECG trace was available for checking. Eighty-five patients received lignocaine. On three occasions, atrial fibrillatation or supraventricular tachycardia was mistaken for ventricular tachycardia. There was also one important error — fortunately without ill effect, when lignocaine was given to a patient with a slow idioventricular rhythm. In terms of ECG abnormality 111 of 212 patients were considered to have responded wholly or partly to their drugs, but we have no means of judging the clinical value of these responses. Atropine was never followed by ventricular fibrillation, though a causal relationship has been suggested by some workers.

The principal functions of a coronary ambulance system are to facilitate admission to hospital by eliminating unnecessary delays and to eliminate death from primary ventricular fibrillation in transit. It is impossible to know whether or not our drug therapy ever prevents ventricular fibrillation which sometimes occurs while patients are being moved. Certainly we expect prompt and efficient defibrillation under these circumstances. There was one case during the first year of our experience (1971) in which defibrillation took four minutes, and the patient did not survive. There, error was in the training; I had told the ambulancemen very emphatically to make absolutely certain that the patient was dead before giving a shock. In stressing that there must be no sign of life, I did not allow for the convulsive movements, nor for the irregular gasping respiratory efforts which can continue long after circulatory arrest. Consequently the ambulanceman was uncertain about defibrillation until the patient had stopped breathing and it was then too late to be successful. Fortunately this very early experience has not been repeated. In the only two patients who have died with

Table 1: Drug Administration by Ambulancemen 1974-5

	No. Patients	Indications Correct	Apparently 'Beneficial' ECG Response
Atropine	127	126 (+ 1 unknown)	56
Lignocaine	85	81	55
Totals	212	207 (?+1)	111

ventricular fibrillation during transit in 1974-5, the dysrhythmia accompanied profound cardiogenic shock and I am satisfied that no treatment could have been successful.

Results of Attempted Resuscitation

Table 2 shows the overall results of attempted resuscitation in 1974 and 1975. Forty-seven were in asystole when first seen and none survived. Another 160 had ventricular fibrillation, all but thirteen of whom were found with this dysrhythmia. Coordinated rhythm was restored at least transiently in sixty-six patients. Twenty-seven survived to leave hospital, including sixteen who had been in fibrillation when first seen by the ambulance attendants.

The use of portable equipment in the last 2½ years has modified our concepts of the role of out-of-hospital resuscitation. Until 1974 we had no success in patients already in ventricular fibrillation when the ambulance arrived. Since then the emphasis has changed completely; we now *expect* most to be in this category. Our recent experience is remarkable in that most of our survivors have had complete respiratory arrest before resuscitation was initiated, and some had dilated pupils. Collapse and apparent death have usually preceded '999' calls for an ambulance in these cases; times under such circumstances can rarely be obtained accurately, but intervals of five to seven minutes seem relatively common. We cannot tell of course whether or not some patients had a limited circulation before the first ECG record showed ventricular fibrillation.   The following case report illustrates an example of pre-hospital resuscitation:

Table 2: Results of Attempted Resuscitation 1974-5

	From Asystole	From Ventricular Fibrillation
Attempts at resuscitation	47	160
Coordinated rhythm restored	0	66
Survived to leave hospital	0	27*

*Includes sixteen patients who were already in ventricular fibrillation when first seen by ambulancemen.

Mr F.M. (age fifty-one years) complained of pain in the left shoulder while playing golf. He decided to walk back to the clubhouse in the belief that he had pulled a muscle, leaving his companions to continue their game. Subsequently another group of golfers noticed a trolley apparently unattended on the seventeenth fairway. As they approached they saw a figure lying prone, and ran to investigate. Mr F.M. was found unconscious, grey, apnoeic, and with dilated pupils (a sign with which one of the observers was familiar). One golfer had read of external massage and attempted it while colleagues ran to a nearby house to telephone for help. A resuscitation ambulance arrived (via the eighteenth and seventeenth fairways!) about seven minutes after the patient had been found, and an unknown time after he had collapsed. The ambulancemen confirmed that the patient was cyanosed and pulseless; he was having effective massage but no ventilation save for a few spontaneous gasps. The oscilloscope showed coarse ventricular fibrillation. One shock at 400 Joules led to asystole; massage and ventilation were continued. Ventricular tachycardia supervened with return of a palpable pulse approximately three minutes after the DC shock. The patient's colour improved and spontaneous breathing returned. The heart rhythm slowed and idioventricular rhythm responded to atropine with return of sinus tachycardia. The patient was electively ventilated in hospital. He regained consciousness the following day and returned to work after about four months.

Freezing conditions may have protected the patient from the effects of anoxia, but his recovery was nevertheless a testimony to the value of even unskilled cardiac compression. Other resuscitations have been equally remarkable; many have necessitated multiple shocks as well as drug administration and often intubation for effective ventilation.

The Value of the Scheme

Our better results since 1974 may be due in part to an increased awareness within the community of what should be done when someone collapses. The coronary ambulances are well known and popular. We can cite as evidence that during two weeks of 1974, nearly 10,000 people signed a petition to retain the ambulances which they believed (incorrectly) were threatened by the Area Health Authority. There is usually little delay before a '999' call and often some attempt is made at first aid. Unfortunately, an almost insignificant proportion of the general public has had instruction in external cardiac massage and only rarely has this been performed effectively before arrival of the ambulance. The much better results of out-of-hospital resuscitation reported from Seattle have been achieved by a massive programme of public education which we are only now beginning to emulate and, initially at least, to a very limited extent.

The dangers of moving patients after infarction are often emphasised but as far as short distances are concerned they may be overrated. Pronounced increases in heart rate are said to occur. We attempted to examine those who did not subsequently show evidence of infarction and patients who had been given drugs which could affect heart rate; we had data from only twenty-eight. The work was carried out by Roger Hawkes who was spending time with us as a medical student. He made an important contribution at a time when our difficulties after reorganisation were at their greatest. R-R intervals were obtained on a histogram by playing the tapes through a dysrhythmia computer. The first movement of patients and the start and completion of ambulance journeys were marked by coded signals. Unfortunately, for logistic reasons, the tapes were not usually running continuously during the whole period of transfer into the ambulance, but the data are otherwise complete. We have taken as 100 per cent the heart rate of the patient before he was moved. The averaged heart rate as a result of moving into the ambulance and the peak rates during the journey were almost identical to the averaged initial rates, though at the time of arrival within the coronary care unit the readings were slightly slower (Figure 3). That is not to say that *some* people do not get an increase in heart rate because they do, but the changes occurred in both directions and were not great so that differences averaged out. We intend to make a more detailed study along similar lines.

We conducted a poll of the general practitioners in the area to assess their opinion of the service provided by the resuscitation ambulances. A complicated questionnaire was sent to 141 practitioners and we received 129 replies (92 per cent), which seemed a good response, with 126 in favour of the system, two 'don't knows' and one who said it was a 'stupid gimmick'. The only frequently expressed doubt concerned the safety of intubation by ambulancemen, but we have been very reassured by our experience to date.

I think most would accept that a coronary ambulance or resuscitation ambulance system is of value. It can to a small degree reduce fatality, particularly by enabling patients to reach hospital quickly and safely, but also by providing an effective means of

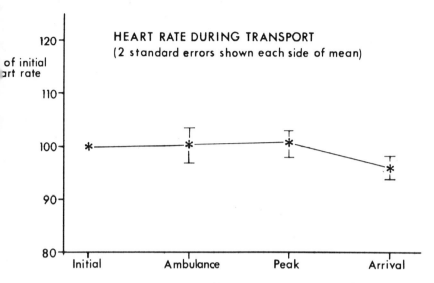

Figure 3   Average heart rate response in 28 patients with myocardial infarction
as a result of movement to an ambulance and journey to hospital. Changes in
rate were expressed as a percentage of the rate first observed before the
patient was moved. None of this group was treated with atropine or lignocaine.

resuscitation for some people who collapse without warning. There are
other less obvious benefits, not least of which is the remarkable extent
to which the standard of care is improved for all patients carried by
the ambulances; this effect is not limited to the attendants who have
undergone special training. We accept that the best results can be
achieved by skilled medical attendants; it would be foolish to pretend
that ambulancemen can resuscitate more effectively than doctors with
special experience in this field. But it is not always possible to have
resuscitation ambulances manned by skilled medical attendants. In
Brighton we have adopted a compromise which is, I believe, a useful
one and one which provides some real benefits for the community.

Notes

1. Pantridge, J.F. and Geddes, J.S., 'A Mobile Intensive Care Unit in the Management of Myocardial Infarction', *Lancet,* 1967, 2, 271.
2. Cobb, L.A. *et al.,* 'Resuscitation from Out-of-Hospital Ventricular Fibrillation, Four Years Follow Up', *Circulation,* 1975, Supplement No.3, 223.
3. Gearty, G.F., *et al.,* 'Pre-Hospital Coronary Care Service', *British Medical Journal,* 1971, 3, 33.
4. White, N.M. *et al.,* 'Mobile Coronary Care Provided by Ambulance Personnel', *British Medical Journal,* 1973, 3, 618.
5. Briggs, R.S. *et al.,* 'The Brighton Resuscitation Ambulances: A Continuing Experiment in Pre-hospital Care by Ambulance Staff', *British Medical Journal,* 1976, 2, 1161.

9 CORONARY CARE IN THE INDUSTRIAL WORK PLACE

Dr Robert Mayes

The provision of primary coronary care in the industrial environment is a logical extension to care in the community at large. Industrial medicine is increasing in extent and importance, and many industries now have extensive and sophisticated medical departments which are equipped to deal quickly and effectively with acute industrial emergencies. Acute myocardial infarction (AMI) is the commonest non-industrial emergency they will encounter, and it would seem reasonable that they should be equipped to deal with it. This chapter describes the primary care given by the medical team of a large industrial complex to a work force of over 12,000.

The medical department concerned is long established and provides a service for a number of high-risk chemical plants situated on a site covering two square miles, as well as two refineries and a number of smaller plants seven miles away. The department is situated in a central position on the site, which is provided with a good road system and easy access to the plants. The nature of the chemical plants means, however, that there are problems with rescue and movement of patients. The total work force employed is in excess of 12,000, of which less than 5 per cent are women. Approximately 40 per cent are administrative, management or supervisory staff and the remaining 60 per cent are made up of craftsmen, process workers and labourers of one kind or another. Fifty-five per cent are aged forty or over, which means that more than 6,000 men can be considered at risk of AMI. It is estimated that between fifteen and twenty cases of myocardial infarction occur on the site each year.

The department is staffed by three full-time medical officers, all of whom have had experience in general practice. In addition to their routine work they provide twenty-four-hour emergency cover. During normal working hours one doctor is always present in the building and immediately available, while during the silent hours an on-call rota is operated with one doctor always on call. The nursing staff include eighteen State Registered Nursing Officers as well as five medical orderlies, who are usually forces-trained, and as well as acting as ambulance drivers they are able to assist in resuscitation and treatment.

The emergency cover is maintained over the twenty-four hours on a three-shift system, each shift consisting of two Nursing Officers and an orderly, although during normal working hours this is augmented by the day staff.

There are six ambulances on the site, two of which are always stationed at the central medical department for emergency use. The ambulances are converted Cortina Estate cars which carry a single stretcher and are fully equipped for resuscitation and emergency treatment. They are usually driven by an orderly, who is accompanied by a Nursing Officer, but every Nursing Officer is expected to be able to drive an ambulance if needed.

The main medical department was built sixteen years ago and comprises the ground floor of an office block in a central position on the site. Apart from the normal consulting rooms and treatment facilities, it includes a six-bed emergency ward. One of these beds has been reserved for primary coronary care and is equipped with piped oxygen, a monitor and ECG recorder. With it is a special drug trolley containing readily available supplies of heroin, atropine, lignocaine, digoxin, frusemide, practolol, sodium bicarbonate and diazepam. All the Nursing Officers are trained in the taking of electrocardiographs (ECG) and the use of the monitor. They have been instructed in reading ECGs, recognising abnormalities and dysrhythmias, and in the indications for the use of the defibrillator. Defibrillation is carried out under medical supervision whenever possible, but the Nursing Officer is expected to be able to use the defibrillator in the doctors' absence if she considers it necessary.

Because of the high risk of toxic gas release and explosion associated with chemical production, the emergency procedure on the site is highly organised. Apart from a priority emergency number on the internal telephone system, based on the '999' call, there is an audible alarm and a direct line from the emergency control centre to the medical department. Following the receipt of an emergency call, the Cortina ambulance and Nursing Officer can be at the scene of the incident within three to four minutes, and the patient back at the medical centre within a further five minutes. This compares favourably with even the best organised ambulance service; the local ambulance cannot guarantee to reach the site within fifteen minutes. On receiving the emergency call, the works ambulance sets out, the doctor on duty is informed and the ward prepared to receive the patient. On arrival on the ward, the patient is immediately monitored and an ECG recording taken. Treatment is commenced as indicated and the local hospital coronary care unit is informed.

The patient's condition is stabilised and he is monitored and kept under continuous observation for at least two hours. In cases of difficulty, advice is sought from the hospital, and the local consultant physician is prepared to come to the site if required. When the patient's condition is thought to be satisfactory, he is transferred by the Cortina ambulance to the hospital coronary care unit, accompanied by the doctor and one of the Nursing Officers. It is the policy of the department to admit all cases of myocardial infarction to the hospital for further observation, rather than send them home to the care of their family doctor.

The establishment of the primary coronary care unit in the medical department followed discussion with local consultant physicians, after a survey had been carried out in the cases of myocardial infarction occurring on the site in the period 1957 to 1966. This showed that there were 121 cases recorded. Of these: 43 were dead on arrival at the department; 12 died in the department; 8 died later in hospital; 58 survived. Accurate figures have not been kept since then, but in 1975 there were fifteen cases recorded of which: 3 were dead on arrival; 1 died later in hospital; 2 were defibrillated and survived; 9 survived without defibrillation. The two patients who required defibrillation both recovered completely and have now returned to their normal work.

The first case was a foreman, aged fifty-four, who walked into the department complaining that he had felt some pain in his chest over the preceding three hours. His condition was good when examined, his pulse 70 regular, BP 140/90 and normal heart sounds. An ECG was taken which showed evidence of an anterior infarction. Within a few minutes he developed ventricular fibrillation, was defibrillated and his rhythm was restored to normal. He was transferred to the hospital coronary care unit where he made an uneventful recovery and returned to his normal employment after four months.

The second case was a supervisor, again aged fifty-four, who collapsed suddenly with severe chest pain. On admission to the department he was in severe shock and almost immediately went into ventricular fibrillation. He was successfully defibrillated but his rhythm remained very unstable. The hospital was informed and on the advice of the consultant he was transferred to the coronary care unit where a pacemaker was inserted. The patient has now recovered completely and has returned to his normal employment.

There is no doubt that this service can be criticised, and it needs to be improved in the light of more modern views on treatment. It is apparent that primary care needs to be supplied to the patient at the earliest possible moment and this means carrying mobile equipment and trained staff to the patient, not transporting the patient to the equipment. We hope that a mobile monitor and defibrillator will be provided for use at the scene of the incident. It is also hoped that there will be full cooperation with the new coronary care car which will be in operation from the hospital in the very near future. It should then be possible continuously to monitor and resuscitate a patient who has had a myocardial infarction, beginning within a few minutes of the time that he develops a pain in his chest; first by the works emergency service and then by the hospital coronary care team.

We have shown that primary coronary care can be carried out successfully in the industrial environment. There are possibly many other factories and industrial health centres supplying similar facilities and there are descriptions of life support units provided by industry in America. The intention is not to replace the community or hospital services but to augment them and to work in cooperation with them. The industrial medical service stands in the forefront of emergency care and because of the nature of its work, especially in the high risk areas, is organised to treat emergencies rapidly and effectively. Coronary thrombosis is such an emergency and requires equal speed and efficiency.

10 PRIMARY CARE AFTER MYOCARDIAL INFARCTION: COMMUNITY SERVICES PROVIDED BY GENERAL PRACTITIONERS

Introduction

At the time of the National Workshop on Coronary Care in the Community in 1976, only three groups of general practitioners in Britain were known to be operating or planning to provide a mobile coronary care unit, using monitors and defibrillators. There may have been others but national advertising by various means failed to reveal them.

By the time of the Workshop, Dr Brian Jones and his colleagues in Worsley near Manchester had much valuable experience and advice to offer. Their scheme was notable in that they had succeeded in cutting across the usual practice barriers, to provide a community service. Dr Brian Sproule of Coldstream had the advantage of a cottage hospital and full-time nursing cover. Dr Clifford Cowley and his partners in Ramsey cared for all the patients in the north end of the Isle of Man and also had a cottage hospital. They were just beginning their scheme and were reluctant to appear in print at such an early stage. Nevertheless, their early experience and difficulties, together with the other reports, may be of value to those who contemplate providing such a service.

Each author describes how groups of local doctors have assessed the needs of the community, and applied their resources in the most effective way possible. Their patients have responded by providing money for equipment. There is further discussion in Chapter 12 about whether such developments are necessary and the importance of careful monitoring of results.

I WORSLEY

Dr Brian Jones

The Worsley Community Coronary Care Team was a development of
the Coronary Care Service based at Hope Hospital, Salford, a district
general hospital serving a population of nearly 300,000 people. This
hospital had instituted a coronary care unit in the early days of the
development of these units when the physicians in the area became
aware of the nature of coronary care and the consequences of cardiac
arrest. The unit started in a small way with two monitored beds and a
specially detailed staff trained in giving coronary care. It was made
possible by voluntary contributions from the local people. In Salford
this impetus originated in general practice and it is of interest that the
more recent thoughts on coronary care are moving towards activities
in the community based on general practice.

The Hospital Based Coronary Care System

The most important principle in the development of the coronary care
unit was the recognition that, after a cardiac arrest, the heart function
could be restored if this were done within the critical four-minute
period during which the brain could survive, but a prerequisite was the
presence of the necessary countershock defibrillator equipment and
staff skilled in using it. It was recognised that such a dysrhythmic arrest
could happen at any time during the days after the acute ischaemic
incident and logically such patients were better cared for with
continuous monitoring by people skilled in the necessary techniques of
recognition of dysrhythmia and its degeneration. Within a short space
of time six beds were provided in a specially designed department
manned by specially trained nursing staff with two senior house officers
designated to the unit.

Mobile Coronary Care Unit

Following the development of the mobile coronary care unit by
Professor Pantridge in Belfast, a similar unit was begun in Salford. From
the beginning general practitioners were involved in the discussions of
the coronary care programme and the debates and arguments about it.
They recognised that a patient with acute myocardial ischaemia could
arrest before the arrival of the team from the parent coronary care unit.

So the general practitioners were invited to a series of lectures on coronary care and the management of cardiac arrest. It was suggested that they should respond promptly to any request from a patient who presented with the features of acute myocardial ischaemia. They were asked to monitor the heart rate and rhythm by continually palpating the pulse, to relieve pain and anxiety and, in the event of arrest, to ventilate the patient and perform closed chest cardiac massage. All general practitioners were issued with an Ambu bag attached to a Brooke airway, and training sessions using the resuscit-Annie dummy were given.

Several general practitioners had experience of maintaining a circulation whilst awaiting the arrival of the mobile coronary care unit, and there were several instances of successful defibrillation performed by general practitioners using cardiac massage and ventilation prior to the arrival of the defibrillator.

Such activity led to the admission to the district general hospital of far more cases of acute myocardial ischaemia than before and the pattern of general practitioner care of coronary thrombosis changed in a matter of weeks. Whereas formerly a great number of patients were kept at home, now they were all admitted to the district general hospital through the coronary care unit and the six beds were nearly always occupied. Some were decanted into the general wards of the hospital and later to a follow-up ward. This new admission policy and pattern of care put a great strain on the beds in the district general hospital. Many cases entered monitored care and had a completely uneventful passage into a fourteen-day convalescent period in the follow-up ward and were then discharged. It was recognised that it was impossible to differentiate between those who would recover uneventfully and those who would arrest. Herein was the dilemma of care; it was impossible to ignore the conclusion that some patients could arrest at home where monitoring and resuscitation were impossible within the four minute period.

It was also recognised that the mean time of application of care via the mobile unit was about four and a half hours. We knew that arrest was most likely within the first hour, probably within the first half hour. Consequently the mobile coronary care unit was reaching only about half the cases who would arrest, as well as the 50 per cent of the total cases who would have an uneventful experience. The hospital-based coronary care unit was unable to offer a direct callout from the public for the monitored resuscitation service, which led to long delays. By the time the patient, or those in attendance, had decided that he was

suffering from a serious coronary incident and called the general
practitioner (who was often not instantly available), at least an hour
had elapsed. From our two years experience of monitoring we found
it unusual for calls to come within the first hour. (General practitioners
at that time were, and still are, largely unavailable on bleep or radio
callout.)

Trained Ambulance Personnel

An attempt was made to shorten this delay by using trained ambulance
personnel who answered '999' calls to such incidents. The ambulance
men were trained in the recognition of the ischaemic attack and in
monitoring patients by palpation of the pulse, together with
ventilation and cardiac massage if necessary while waiting for the
mobile coronary care unit to arrive. They were asked not to bring the
patient in by ordinary ambulance. Many of these ambulance drivers
had previous experience of moving such patients who died during
transfer to hospital.

A commercial traveller owes his life to the fact that an ambulance crew
attending a '999' call to a shop in the area, recognised that it was an
acute myocardial ischaemic attack and, instead of putting him into
their ambulance they called the mobile coronary care unit. When the unit
arrived the patient was in sinus rhythm and while an electrocardiograph
was being done he went unheralded into ventricular fibrillation
and was promptly defibrillated. He made an uneventful recovery.

The General-Practitioner-Based Mobile Coronary Care Unit

In an attempt to apply care within the early hours, preferably as soon
as possible after the onset of an acute myocardial ischaemic attack, it
was decided to form a team of general practitioners in Worsley and
equip it with the necessary monitoring and resuscitation equipment.

Training

The doctors were trained in the recognition of the acute myocardial
ischaemic attack, the intravenous use of drugs, how to stabilise the
heart rate and rhythm and in the techniques of defibrillation if there
was a cardiac arrest. Training sessions were held at fortnightly intervals
throughout the winter of 1973-4 and they were attended by many more
general practitioners than the eight who eventually formed the team.
The team members had further training in a coronary care unit using
special equipment to teach the recognition of rate and rhythm

disturbances on a monitorscope and also defibrillation techniques.

Equipment

Money for the necessary equipment was raised by voluntary subscription. The equipment purchased was a robust portable monitorscope by Simonsen and Weel, which was large and heavy but gave a clear non-fading image and had a long-capacity rechargeable battery, a Pantridge defibrillator with two rechargeable batteries and an electrocardiograph. A bag was equipped with intravenous canulae and syringes, sphygmomanometer, tourniquet and the necessary drugs. This bulky and heavy equipment was housed in a small van which was used by the team member on call as his vehicle for the day. He carried a bleep, the van was equipped with a radio and so he was available if a call came to the radio controller from the general public. He was able to respond to a call immediately and could monitor and resuscitate a patient within minutes of callout. The equipment was carried in a van because it was too bulky and heavy to be transferred from one doctor's car to another. This equipment was chosen and purchased three years ago. It is now being replaced by much lighter, more compact combined equipment which will make the use of an expensive separate van unnecessary.

Education of the Public

The appeal for money to buy equipment was coupled with gentle education and was a public relations exercise aimed at getting patients to call early in order that care could be applied as soon as possible. There was some concern that the necessary education of the public in the need for the early callout would lead to excessive anxiety and an uncontrollable demand for the service. The Department of Psychology at the University of Manchester was consulted and it was decided that such a reaction on the part of the public was unlikely. Possibly people would take little notice of such advice but if they did they would only remember it when the incident actually occurred and this is what happened. The public was informed by leaflet saying that in the event of anyone having a severe pain across the chest which they had never had before (or if they were used to having angina and it was not relieved by the use of their Gly. Trinitrin tablets) they should call the unit by telephoning a special number. They were informed that a team would visit them and decide whether they needed further care. The leaflet also reminded the public that this was a voluntary service operated by general practitioners and that in the event of it not being possible at times to provide such a service, then the radio operator receiving the call would institute conventional care systems. This was included because it was recognised that the equipment would not always be serviceable, that the vehicle would not be necessarily always on the road and that at holiday times it might not be possible to keep a full team available.

The Team went into action on 1 April 1974 and on average attends three calls per week, half the expected incidence for such a community.

Procedure

The team member carries the monitorscope and the bag containing the intravenous equipment and drugs to the patient. He asks someone else to bring the electrocardiograph and the defibrillator from the vehicle. The first object is to stabilise the rate and rhythm with a view to preventing cardiac arrest. The patient's pain and anxiety are first of all relieved with a strong analgesic of the doctor's own choice: in my case this is intravenous diamorphine (heroin). All drugs are given intravenously because the desired effects can be attained by titration, enabling the smallest dose of a drug to be given. The effect is quickest by the intravenous route and speed of action is valuable since dysrhythmia may occur. I dissolve the heroin in prochlorperazine (stemetil). (Freeze-dried diamorphine is necessary as this does not degenerate.) Several authorities have been consulted as to the possible adverse effect of dissolving freeze-dried diamorphine in prochlorperazine and none are known. Another reason for using the intravenous technique in preference to intramuscular routes is the enzymes liberated from the muscular site of injection are not going to complicate enzyme surveys during the next few days. All drugs are given by an intravenous canula (the small butterfly canula is used by us) secured in position with sellotape. Having relieved the patient's pain and anxiety (intravenous diazepam (valium) is sometimes used where anxiety persists after pain relief) attention is given, and indeed is given throughout, to observation of the scope which has been attached to the patient from the doctor's arrival. In the event of a bradycardia below 50 per minute, doses of 0.3 mg of atropine are given at three-minute intervals until the rate is brought up to 70. A tachycardia in excess of 90 per minute or the presence of ventricular extrasystoles is treated by intravenous lignocaine by some members. Beta blockade may be preferred if there is no contraindication such as bronchospasm, history of bronchospasm, heart failure, heart block or the presence in the room of broncho dilator drugs and aerosols. Practolol is preferred since it is cardio protective; it may have the effect of preventing further catechol amine release and the outpouring of free fatty acids. Practolol (10 mg) is given slowly and its effect observed for ten minutes; a bradycardia is likely to follow and intravenous atropine may be necessary. In the event of cardiac failure, jugular venous filling, basal crepitations or triple rhythms, then intravenous frusemide (lasix) is given. Cardiac glycosides are never used in the acute attack. Oxygen is carried but has been used rarely.

The team member enters the identification details of the patient and the name of the patient's own general practitioner on the data retrieval from, together with the estimated time of onset of the ischaemic incident, the time when the patient called for care and the time care was applied. He records the initial blood pressure, pulse rate and rhythm, clinical findings and the care given, on the time scale down the right side of the form which gives a list of possible rate and rhythm disturbances. He enters the electrocardiographic findings together with observations of the scope, the drugs used and their effect.

Further Care

During this control programme a decision is made as to the future care of the patient. Patients are not moved before stabilisation. It has been the policy of the coronary care unit to admit all patients who were considered potentially dysrhythmic within forty-eight hours of the onset of the incident. My own present policy is that when it is more than six hours since the onset of the attack and there is no further discomfort or distress, if the rate and rhythm are stable and there has been no disturbance of rate and rhythm during this initial monitoring, then these cases may be offered home care if it is acceptable to the patient and the relatives. However, if a patient comes under care in less than six hours then it is probably necessary to admit him for continued monitoring. Statistically we are led to believe that dysrhythmia and arrest are possible, although less likely, within the following forty-eight hours and certainly, where rate and rhythm disturbances have been observed in those early hours, arrest is a possibility. However, the findings of the Teesside Coronary Survey[1] and of the Mather survey in Bristol[2] suggest that, given a stable situation, a patient with a recent ischaemia has a better chance of survival if left at home than if he is moved to a general ward. However, where a decision is made to keep the patient at home a calculated risk is undoubtedly taken because if an unheralded dysrhythmia degenerates into ventricular fibrillation or arrest, there is little possibility of resuscitation. Under these circumstances visits to the patient can only elicit the development of heart failure or benign dysrhythmias. In the absence of heart failure such patients should be given antidysrhythmic therapy, either a beta blocker or mexiletine hydrochlor (mexitil) by mouth.

Notes

1. Colling, W.A. *et al.,* 'Teesside Coronary Survey: An Epidemiological Study of Acute Attacks of Myocardial Infarction', *British Medical Journal,* 1976, 2, 1169-72.
2. Mather, H.G. *et al.,* 'Myocardial Infarction. A Comparison between Home and Hospital Care for Patients', *British Medical Journal,* 1976, 1, 925-9.

II   RAMSEY, ISLE OF MAN

Dr Clifford Cowley

The Ramsey group practice in the Isle of Man is unique in many ways. The geographical position of such a well-defined practice area with a relatively static population, enables us to keep fairly reliable long-term statistics. The practice covers the northern two fifths of the island and is roughly in the shape of a triangle, two sides of which are formed by the sea and the base by a sparsely populated range of hills.

The practice operates principally from a group practice centre in the grounds of a well-equipped small hospital in Ramsey, a seaside market town, population 6,000, about halfway down the eastern side of the triangle. There is also a branch surgery in Kirk Michael near the base of the western side of the triangle. The practice cares for approximately 10,800 patients. The nearest coronary care unit is in Douglas, sixteen miles away, and is used only rarely.

For some years we believed that much of the published data for deaths following acute myocardial infarction (AMI) seemed to be higher in other communities than ours. Cases could not occur without our knowledge since we know of every death and every AMI in our community. We knew that impressions can be misleading; as golfers we always appear to be playing well until we start to keep the score. We were greatly stimulated by talks from Dr Colling and Professor Pantridge in 1974 and by a visit to Dr Jones in Manchester, and we decided to endeavour to improve our own treatment of the AMI and also to record the incidence of myocardial infarction and sudden death resulting from coronary heart disease, in the patients of the Ramsey group practice. We were aware that it was essential to get to the patients with the appropriate equipment and drugs as quickly as possible, but that it was impossible for us to equip a coronary ambulance and coronary care unit on Professor Pantridge's scale, partly because we were feeling our way but largely on consideration of cost.

Although we adopted much of Dr Jones' system, we decided that a coronary van would be unsuitable for our practice. Over £2,000 needed to purchase the necessary equipment was raised within three months, chiefly by the local branch of the Manx Variety Club, the local Round Table and one generous donor.

The Ramsey Scheme

Each doctor has a radio telephone in his car and carries the necessary drugs all the time. The portable ECG and monitor, defibrillator and oxygen, are sited in the local hospital, easily available for collection by the patient's doctor or the doctor most readily available. If this is not possible the equipment can be sent out by ambulance car or by one of the secretaries.

This system does have its faults and on two or three occasions the equipment has not arrived in time. However, in 37 cases out of 42 a doctor has reached the patient within 20 minutes of a call and most of these were within 15 minutes.

The big delay factor is the time between the onset of symptoms and the call to the group practice, but we decided not to issue the detailed instructions used in Worsley. We have not changed our view that this would cause more anxiety in the community than was justifiable.

In order to establish the categories of AMI we were dealing with, we used the modified WHO criteria used in the Teesside survey and described in Chapter 3. Each possible AMI had at least one cardiograph and up to six enzyme samples. Suspected cases of AMI were nursed at home if: (i) two hours after the onset of symptoms the general condition of the patient was good, with a normal BP and pulse rate; (ii) the home conditions were satisfactory; (iii) the home was convenient for daily visits by the GP. If these conditions were not met the patient was admitted to the Ramsey hospital.

Equipment

The equipment used for the early treatment of AMI was as follows:

1 Portable Monitor   ) These are all put on charge at regular
1 Portable Defibrillator   ) intervals whether in use or not.
1 Portable ECG
1 Portable Oxygen
Butterfly needles

If we were starting again we would purchase a *lightweight,* combined monitor/defibrillator — we tend to rely on the monitor rather than the ECG in initial treatment.

Drugs

The main drugs used were:

> Diamorphine 5 mg (heroin) dissolved in prochlorperazine
>   25 mg (Stemetil)
> Sotalol 5 mg (Beta-cardone)
> Atropine 0.6 mg
> Lignocaine 50 mg
> Frusemide 40 mg (Lasix)

The most useful drug in our series has been intravenous heroin dissolved in 25 mg prochlorperazine and used on all patients with pain. A rapid and dramatic improvement in the patient's condition was seen in each case. Atropine has been used on most patients with bradycardia, while Sotalol and Lignocaine have been used on patients with tachycardia and multiple extrasystole. We have been a little unhappy about Sotalol given intravenously, since the first two patients collapsed while being treated for tachycardia and multiple extrasystoles.

Results

Out of the first 33 cases who survived the initial attack, 14 were nursed at home and all survived (8 'definite' and 6 'possible' AMIs). Eighteen were nursed in the Ramsey hospital and 3 of them died (10 'definite' and 8 'possible'). One who had pneumonia and a blood sugar of 500 mg (per cent), was sent to the coronary care unit and he died. During this period there were also six sudden deaths and three patients who died within minutes of the doctor arriving on the scene.

Table 1: Treated Cases

	Category of AMI		Deaths
Home	Definite	8	0
	Possible	6	0
Ramsey Hospital	Definite	10	3
	Possible	8	0
CCU	Definite	1	1
Total		33	4

Statistics are very unreliable when dealing with only 42 cases but, as shown below, they also depend on the criteria used.

Fatality (%)

Fatality of All Cases (including sudden deaths)	31.0%
(Fatality of Definite AMIs	46.4%)

If, however, one excludes six sudden deaths and three early deaths that could not possibly have reached the coronary care unit, then:

Fatality of All Cases	12.1%
(Fatality of Definite AMIs	21.1%)

When all treated cases are considered (alive when first seen), then,

Fatality of All Cases	19.4%
(Fatality of Definite AMIs	31.8%)

Time of Call to General Practitioner

Onset of symptoms to call for general practitioner,

Less than 1 hour	19 cases
Between 1-2 hours	3 cases
More than 2 hours	20 cases

If sudden deaths are excluded then the general practitioner was called to about one third of patients within the first hour.

Time of Death

6 Dead on arrival of GP
1 Died 15 minutes after onset of symptoms
1 Died after ventricular fibrillation (VF) 90 minutes after onset.
  (He was defibrillated but did not survive a massive AMI and died in asystole.)
1 Died 210 minutes after onset (probable VF)
1 Died 12 hours after onset in Asystole
1 Died 19 hours after onset in Asystole
1 Died 38 hours after onset (definite VF)
1 Died 6 weeks after onset (congestive failure)

When this scheme started in 1975, we were approaching a spell of cold weather and we saw so many cases, real and suspect, in a short time, that we began to wonder if we had taken on too big a project. When the warm spell started in the summer of 1976) the numbers dropped so markedly that at one time we went for five weeks without seeing a single case.

Conclusions

It is much too soon to draw any firm conclusions from our very early results but already it appears that the patients who survive the initial attack are likely to do well at home and reasonably well in the Ramsey hospital. The main problem is to reach the patient earlier and prevent early death. With this in mind, some of the problems to overcome include: (i) earlier call; (ii) a more efficient way of getting the equipment to the bedside; (iii) the need for more equipment (ideally a lightweight monitor/defibrillator for each doctor); (iv) improved confidence in the use of betablocking drugs; (v) more involvement of the nursing staff and ambulance men; (vi) dealing with a collapsed patient virtually single-handed, even with sophisticated equipment.

The greatest and most obvious benefit so far is probably to the doctors, in that our project has given us a great deal of interest and knowledge of a disease which is probably the most serious that we encounter. Whatever the final statistics will prove to be, this increased interest and knowledge can not be anything but beneficial to our patients.

We hope to publish our results in about three years' time (1979).

III   COLDSTREAM

Dr Brian Sproule

My practice is situated in a rural area on the Scottish-English
border with the nearest general hospital thirty-five miles away and
coronary care unit fifty miles away. The ambulance journeys to these
hospitals take forty-five and sixty minutes respectively. In the centre
of the practice is a general practitioner hospital for general medical and
geriatric cases, and a well-equipped emergency and outpatient room.

Until 1974 no primary care was available to a patient other than
general measures for relief of pain, and an assessment was made as to
the patient's fitness to undertake the journey by ambulance to the
general hospital or coronary care unit. Hospital admission was
considered desirable to achieve cardiac monitoring and better
supervision and nursing. With a patient safely speeding on his way to
a hospital bed his general practitioner would feel satisfied that the
best had been done for him. However, there were aspects which
disturbed many doctors. Patients sometimes developed cardiac arrest
in the presence of a doctor and while cardiac massage and assisted
ventilation could be maintained for considerable periods, without
further assistance these patients died. Patients sometimes died on
their way to hospital when accompanied by a nurse and others often
arrived at a hospital in a state of shock after a prolonged ambulance
journey and failed to survive. Myocardial infarction was considered a
killing disease, both by doctors and the general public, an attitude
which disguised the fact that sufferers were dying unnecessarily.

The years 1974-5 saw a considerable advance in the manufacture
of cardiac monitors and defibrillators, making it possible for the
machines to be portable as well as reliable. This opened up the
possibility of having easily carried packs containing all the essentials
for primary care which could be taken to a patient by a general
practitioner from a central point. In my area the general practitioner
hospital was an obvious choice for such a centre and packs were made
up as follows:

1. A Portable Defibrillator and Monitor

The choice of type of monitor and defibrillator is a personal one, but
I have favoured a combined unit rather than separate machines and also

one that is housed in a robust aluminium case so as to withstand any
knocks during a hurried transit. The paddles can be applied to the
chest for immediate monitoring prior to permanent chest leads being
applied, and are available for defibrillation at any time. The
rechargeable batteries are kept on trickle charge continually in hospital
when not in use. The monitor will run continuously for three hours
and up to forty maximum discharges can be given from one charging.

2. *A Case Containing All the Necessary Apparatus and Drugs*

The case is robust but light and contains three deep drawers. The
contents of each drawer are clearly marked on the outside, and the
drawers can be taken out completely for ease of access when in use.
A detailed list of drugs and apparatus is appended, which is being
continually revised in the light of experience and further advances in
treatment.

Many practitioners and nurses have no practical experience of
intubation so the insertion of any airway with forced ventilation
is recommended. The setting up of an intravenous drip, which may
be desirable, presents a number of practical difficulties to a single-
handed person working in the patient's home, and so this is not
catered for either.

A short booklet is included with details recommended for primary
care. They were originally obtained from the therapeutic protocol of
the coronary care unit at Edinburgh Royal Infirmary, but were scaled
down considerably for use under domiciliary conditions, and because
those using them would be unlikely to be as experienced as a senior
medical registrar. The object of the booklet was to provide help in the
critical situation in which a general practitioner is placed on average
about twelve times a year,[1] and in which he will experience
considerable personal stress. It was also hoped that it would produce a
degree of uniformity amongst the many users. For the same reasons, a
special section has been devoted to advice for nurses.

A form for 'Primary Assessment of Chest Pain' is included which
can be completed by a nurse or doctor on first seeing the patient. All
essential details of the patient are listed under various headings and
can be quickly completed. There is a space provided for progress and
treatment which, if not written down at once, can never be satisfactorily
recalled from memory. If hospital admission of the patient is decided
upon, this assessment form can be used and contains very much more
information than the doctor would be able to include in a normal letter
of referral written under hurried stressful conditions.

3. Portable Oxygen-Giving Equipment with an Ambu Bag Resuscitator

The delivery of oxygen by nasal catheter at 2 litres per minute can do nothing good to an embarrassed myocardium, and suitable apparatus weighing only 4.5 kilograms is obtainable to deliver oxygen at this rate for almost three hours. The oxygen can also be fed into an Ambu bag resuscitator for positive pressure ventilation.

4. An Electrocardiograph

An electrocardiograph is useful, sometimes for myocardial infarction, but more often for dysrhythmias and cardiac irregularities which can not be picked out easily on a monitor screen. However, it is important to emphasise to both doctors and nurses that lack of knowledge in the interpretation of an electrocardiogram should not dissuade them from undertaking primary care. McGuinness[2] has shown that only half the cases of recent myocardial infarction can be diagnosed from the initial ECG, and has rightly emphasised that the early diagnosis of acute myocardial infarction is a clinical one.

Organisation

Reorganisation of attitudes and habits in a practice is necessary so as to ensure that a doctor or nurse with primary care equipment can be at a patient's house within half an hour of receiving a call. Many obstacles have to be overcome, not least the doctor's own inertia. He must re-educate himself to realise that myocardial infarction is a critical situation of life and death in which every minute counts. There are very few similar situations in general practice today when the justification of reaching a case within the shortest time possible is so overwhelming that all other work must be put aside.

The practice receptionist staff have to be trained to question a caller if there is any doubt as to the likelihood of chest pain being a symptom, and to contact a doctor at once if so. Spotting a possible case of myocardial infarction from messages sent to a doctor's surgery can be far from easy as was found in twenty-five consecutive cases seen personally. In fifteen incidences chest pain was mentioned specifically, but in the remaining ten cases many other complaints were mentioned. For two years the exact wording of such messages has been recorded verbatim and some examples are worth quoting: all the cases were found to have had myocardial infarcts.

Case A

Message from the patient's wife: 'He doesn't feel well and has a funny chest again.' The patient was known to have recurrent attacks of chronic bronchitis but also to have been suffering from angina pectoris during the last six months. He was found to have had severe retrosternal pain on rising in the morning, radiating down his left arm and not subsiding after two hours.

Case B

Message from a patient's neighbour: 'She is not feeling well.' No other information was obtainable, despite repeated questioning. The patient was found to be breathless, fibrillating and dyspnoic and in a collapsed state. She died two and a half hours later.

Case C

Message from a patient's wife: 'He has had a bad night, could the doctor look in when he is passing this way?' When seen at midday it was found that the patient had awoken at 2.00 a.m. with severe chest pain, vomiting and sweating, which had subsided after three hours. In addition to an infarct he had a right bundle branch block.

Case D

Message from the patient's wife on a Sunday evening: 'Could you come doctor and bring something for his indigestion?' Patient was found to have severe, persistent left sided pectoral pain radiating down his left arm with sweating and restlessness.

Case E

An evening call from the patient's wife: 'My husband came back from work with severe stomach pains and has vomited.' No other information could be obtained by the doctor himself who received the call. The patient was found to have had severe retrosternal pain for four hours and had vomited once. Only after intensive questioning did he admit reluctantly that he had had a previous infarction.

Indigestion seems to be such a usual presenting symptom that it is safer to regard any out of hours call with this complaint as a likely myocardial infarction until proved otherwise. It is rare for indigestion from gastric causes to be severe enough to warrant a special call to a doctor by a patient.

Three case histories illustrate the primary care equipment in action.

Case F

A call was received at 8.00 a.m. to go to a man with severe chest pain. The primary care equipment was picked up from the general practitioner hospital by the doctor on the way to the patient, arriving at his house at 8.30 a.m. He was aged seventy-six and had had bilateral mid-thigh amputations for severe ischaemic pain from arteriosclerosis. He was in bed but very restless with severe chest pain, vomiting, sweating and pulseless. The blood pressure was 80/60 and heart rate 48 per minute and regular. The paddles of the monitor were applied to his chest to obtain an immediate visual tracing of the cardiac rhythm, while an injection of 'Cyclimorph 15'* was prepared and injected intravenously, providing good pain relief. Permanent chest leads were then applied and connected to the monitor, the paddles being removed but kept in readiness for defibrillation. An electrocardiogram was taken next and this showed an auricular flutter on Lead II, with a severe degree of heart block, ventricular rate of 50 per minute and an inferior infarct on Leads III and AVF. An injection of atropine sulphate 0.6 mg was given by intramuscular injection to raise the cardiac output. Fifteen minutes later the heart rate was 60 per minute, the radial pulse was just palpable and a blood pressure reading of 85/60 was easily taken. An hour after the injection the blood pressure had risen to 100/80, the patient was sleeping peacefully, he was a good colour, not vomiting and no longer shocked.

The situation was explained to the patient's wife, a very level-headed woman and it was emphasised to her the importance of keeping her husband at home rather than subjecting him to any sort of ambulance journey. She agreed with this decision and indeed welcomed the opportunity of being able to nurse him at home, particularly because of the availability of the apparatus to monitor his heart. The monitor was switched off but the chest leads were left in position and the patient was left alone for two hours. After this time he was revisited, the monitor was reconnected and showed a heart rate of 100 per minute, which was regular. His blood pressure was 115/80 and an ECG confirmed that there had been a reversion to normal sinus rhythm with only slight prolongation of the PR interval. His recovery was uneventful thereafter, his wife and the community nurses coping adequately with the necessary nursing care. He was sitting in a chair

---

* Cyclimorph – morphine tartrate 15 mg, cyclizine tartrate 50 mg.

after five days, but, as he was legless, walking involved considerable extra exertion with either prostheses or crutches, and was somewhat slower than normal. However, this was accomplished within three weeks and some six weeks later he was enquiring when he would be fit enough to drive his specially adapted car. Needless to say his morale was very high. This case is quoted as it reciprocates very closely the two cases described by Colling in 1974.[1] With these in mind and the added support of monitoring, with a defibrillator on hand if necessary, it was felt that home care and management was the right treatment for this man. Never at any stage had there been any question of moving him from home, initially because he was too ill and latterly because it was unnecessary.

Case G

A call was received at 2.10 p.m. to go to a man aged fifty-eight who had severe chest pain and was known to have had two previous myocardial infarctions. The primary care equipment was picked up by the doctor on his way to the patient, arriving at the patient's home at 2.35 p.m. He was sitting on a sofa and crying with pain, sweating profusely and shocked. The monitor could not be applied immediately to the patient as he was sitting, but it was thought that the relief of pain was of prime importance. While 'Cyclimorph 15' was being prepared he became unconscious, pulseless and ceased breathing. His shirt was torn open and the paddles applied to his chest confirming ventricular fibrillation. Two shocks of 100 and 200 Joules were given before his heart beat became palpable again. His lungs were inflated twice prior to normal ventilation returning and within five minutes the patient had regained consciousness, apologising for any inconvenience he may have caused. Permanent chest leads were then connected to the monitor, showing a heart rate of 120 per minute with a few extra ventricular complexes. Practolol 10 mg by intravenous injection was given, which reduced the heart rate to 100 per minute. The patient lived on his own and could not be nursed at home, so he was removed by ambulance to the general practitioner hospital ten miles away, the doctor accompanying him on the journey with the monitor still attached to the patient, and all the necessary primary care equipment at hand. This journey was achieved satisfactorily and the patient arrived at the hospital in a reasonable condition. This primary care had been carried out by a doctor single-handed and without any other assistance, and while it was not an ideal situation it was certainly a feasible one.

Once at the general practitioner hospital the help of two nurses became available and the management was therefore easier for the doctor. An ECG showed an extensive anterior infarct with a heart rate of 120 per minute and occasional ventricular complexes. It was decided, as cardiac arrest had occurred, that it would be advisable for this case to be monitored for the next forty-eight hours and transferred to the nearest coronary care unit, although necessitating a journey by ambulance of 50 miles. After an hour it was thought that the patient was fit enough to travel and the journey was started, the patient being accompanied by a doctor and a nurse. Within half an hour and having travelled some twelve miles the patient developed ventricular asystole and required resuscitation by cardiac massage. He now had a complete heart block and the heart stopped at least six times, on each occasion being restarted by cardiac massage but the heart rate becoming slower and slower until finally resuscitation was abandoned.

This death raises the question of the advisability of transporting any case of myocardial infarction for a prolonged distance by ambulance. This was noted initially by Kinlen in 1973,[3] when he found that cases of myocardial infarction admitted to the Oxford hospitals from the rural areas and having had an ambulance journey of over thirty minutes appeared to have a worse prognosis than those from within the city boundary, and this has been mentioned again more recently in 1976 by Acheson and Sanderson.[4]

The patient might have survived had he been left at the general practitioner hospital and not transferred to a coronary care unit. The lack of disturbance may have lessened his chances of subsequently developing ventricular asystole and heart block, but had he developed these in the general practitioner hospital, the measures would have been easier to apply than in an ambulance.

Case H

A call was received at midnight from a man aged sixty-one who had had severe chest pain for one hour. There was a previous history of a myocardial infarction four months earlier with subsequent angina pectoris and hypertension. The primary care equipment was picked up by the doctor on his way to the patient who was found to be apprehensive, sweating slightly and with a heart rate of 40 per minute with a sinus rhythm and slight irregularity with ST changes indicating an inferior infarct. The patient was given diamorphine 5 mg by intravenous injection and atropine sulphate 0.6 mg by intramuscular injection and frusemide 20 mg by intramuscular injection. Within 30 minutes the heart rate had risen to 50 and the patient's general condition had improved considerably. He was monitored for two hours, given a further injection of 'Cyclimorph 15' intravenously prior to being left to sleep for the rest of the night and the monitor disconnected. Next morning there were no signs of congestive failure, the heart rate was 84 per minute and regular with an occasional ventricular complex and a BP of 170/100. The question of hospital admission was discussed with both the patient and his wife, both of them expressing a wish to remain at home, which was considered medically to be the best course in any case as the home conditions were very good. The patient was nursed by his wife and the community nurses and within twenty-four hours he was ambulant to the toilet and sitting in a chair four days later.

Conclusions

These cases illustrate how portable primary care equipment units can be used by a general practitioner for the treatment of myocardial infarction. The concept of primary care pioneered by Pantridge and his Belfast team in 1966[5] and followed by many centres subsequently throughout the world,[6] has always been hospital-based, with a mobile coronary care unit going out into the surrounding area from a coronary care unit of a hospital.[7, 8] These units, however, have to rely upon the initial call coming either from the public (sometimes discouraged) or from general practitioners or community nurses. There must inevitably be a time lag, and the organisational implications of running a mobile coronary care unit are formidable. It is logical therefore to consider primary care to be as much a community problem as a hospital one, and with the necessary apparatus and training it has been shown to be possible for general practitioners and nurses to carry this out satisfactorily. Thus the time before treatment is initiated can be greatly reduced. The treatment becomes available to patients in rural areas far removed from a hospital. The running of the scheme is simplified because treatment is given by the nurses and doctors who usually care for the patient, and it emphasises the advantages of home care[9, 10] and nursing.

Primary care can be defined as covering a period of three hours from the onset of chest pain occurring outside a general hospital, or a longer period to allow for transportation to a hospital. It entails the constant attendance and general care of the patient, the application and interpretation of a cardiac monitor, the correction of gross dysrhythmias and treatment of cardiac arrest if this should occur, and it is carried out by suitably trained nurses and general practitioners. The scheme, as outlined, is adaptable to the needs of many different areas and conditions. The greatest and hardest work required initially is in the organisation, training and coordination of the local doctors and nurses, and the education of the community of the area. This may entail blood, sweat and tears but not, fortunately, money as the scheme has the advantage of being comparatively cheap in both manpower and apparatus.

Appendix: Contents of Primary Care Case

Sphygmomanometer and Stethoscope	1 each
ECG Jelly	1 tube
'Micropore' tape 2 cm.	1 roll
Scissors	1 pair
Vein cannulae	3
Syringes 2, 5 and 20 ml.	5 each
Needles, 19, 21 and 23 G.	10 each
'Medi Swabs'	10
Cotton Wool Balls	1 pack
Primary Assessment Forms	10
Therapeutic booklet	1
Drugs:	
Atropine Sulphate 0.6 mg /1ml	5
Diamorphine 5 mg/1 ml	5
Diazepam 10 mg/2 ml	5
Digoxin (Lanoxin) 0.5 mg/2 ml	5
Frusemide 20 mg/2 ml	5
Lignocaine (Xylocard) 2%/5 ml	5
Lignocaine (Xylocard) 10%/3 ml	3
Phenytoin 250 mg/5 ml	5
Practolol 10 mg/5 ml	5
Sodium Bicarbonate 8.4%/100 ml	2

Addendum

Dr Sproule published a letter in the *British Medical Journal* on 29 January 1977, reporting six cardiac arrests treated during 1976. External cardiac massage and forced ventilation were successful in 2 out of 3 cases and defibrillation once out of a further three cases. He wrote, 'I hope that the figures quoted will persuade general practitioners who may question their own usefulness in treating cardiac arrest that their presence during the first two or three hours after a myocardial infarction can be lifesaving.' (Editor)

Notes

1. Colling, A., 'Home or Hospital Care after Myocardial Infarction. Is This the Right Question?', *British Medical Journal,* 1974, 1, 559-63.
2. McGuinness, J.B., Begg, T.B. and Semple, T., 'First Electrocardiogram in Recent Myocardial Infarction', *British Medical Journal,* 1976, 2, 449-51.
3. Kinlen, L.J., 'Incidence and Presentation of Myocardial Infarction in an English Community', *British Heart Journal,* 1973, 35, 616-22.
4. Acheson, R.M. and Sanderson, C., 'Myocardial Infarction: Home and Hospital Treatment', *British Medical Journal,* 1976, 2, 105.
5. Pantridge, J.F. and Geddes, J.S., 'A Mobile Intensive Care Unit in the Management of Myocardial Infarction', *Lancet,* 1967, II, 271.
6. Pantridge, J.F. *et al., The Acute Coronary Attack,* pp.130-1. Pitman Medical Publication, 1975.
7. Julian, D.G., 'Coronary Care and the Community', *Annals of Internal Medicine* 1968, 69, 607.
8. Nixon, P.G.F., 'Coronary Care Units and the Community. Flying Squad Services,' in *Acute Myocardial Infarction,* p.318. (Editors Julian, D.G. and Oliver, M.F.), London, 1968.
9. Colling, A. *et al.,* 'Teesside Coronary Survey: An Epidemiological Study of Acute Attacks of Myocardial Infarction', *British Medical Journal,* 1976, 2, 1169-72.
10. Mather, H.G. *at al.,* 'Myocardial Infarction: A Comparison between Home and Hospital Care for Patients', *British Medical Journal,* 1976, 1, 925-9.

PART THREE   GUIDE LINES
FOR GENERAL PRACTITIONERS

11 GUIDE LINES FOR PRIMARY CARE AFTER MYOCARDIAL INFARCTION

In the National Workshop on Coronary Care in 1976, groups of general practitioners from different areas discussed their role in the management of cases of acute myocardial infarction. The secretary of each group has summarised their conclusions in this chapter. Inevitably there are differences in emphasis, reflecting the experience of the members who were present and the special knowledge of those reporting.

INTRODUCTION
Dr Aubrey Colling

Transition Period

As a result of community surveys and individual studies such as those described earlier, we are now in a more favourable position to formulate guidelines for primary care after myocardial infarction. We are now in a transitional period in which the attitudes of the profession and the public are changing. Young practitioners are aware of many of the facts and figures but have been wary of treating patients at home because of possible recrimination if they died unexpectedly. The educated public expects intensive care and may be rather alarmed by the prospect of treatment at home. There are those, such as Professor Julian (Chapter 6) who warn that the true benefit to an individual patient in a coronary care unit may be lost in the statistics which appear to indicate the superiority of home care for those coming under care after two or three hours. On the other hand, if patients are sent to hospital they sometimes die during transit unless they are monitored adequately and can be resuscitated if arrest occurs. In Belfast[1] death during transfer to hospital has been largely eliminated by the mobile coronary care unit, hence any loss of life in this period of care is no longer acceptable.

The truth lies somewhere amidst all these statistics. Perhaps it will be easier to discover, both for general practitioners and hospital physicians (and the public), if it is searched for on a community basis.

Some patients clearly do very well at home, others require hospital care. It must be understood that there is no certain way of differentiating those who will arrest from those who will not. If patients are transferred to hospital then they must be monitored. If this is not possible then there is considerable risk to the patient which the referring doctor must include in his calculations. Home and hospital care are complementary and can only be understood on this basis.

Some general recommendations are shown in Figure 1. These are guidelines only and are not meant to be strict criteria. Each doctor must look at the facilities in his own area and decide what is appropriate. For example, Dr Sproule (Chapter 10) in Coldstream is fifty miles from the nearest coronary care unit (CCU) and will have different guidelines from those who practice within one or two miles of a CCU. To focus on these differences each type of geographical area is discussed later in this chapter in relation to the hospital facilities available. Is there a coronary ambulance and a CCU? How far is this patient away from the CCU? The general practitioner should not assume that the conditions existing in his local CCU are as good as those in highly specialised units described in the journals. Each general practitioner should decide on a policy and carry it out with full conviction.

Simple Treatment

Many general practitioners are unnecessarily worried by the complexities of modern coronary care. However, the results from Teesside and Bristol have shown that doctors were already achieving good results without any special training. The question is, can they improve them?

The most important points in treatment, without any doubt, are getting quickly to the patient and relieving pain adequately. There is evidence that with good practice organisation, general practitioners can usually reach patients quicker than hospital-based ambulances and vans. General practitioners underrate the service they give, yet it is now believed that many dysrhythmias can be prevented and even reversed by analgesia alone. 'But', the worried doctor argues, 'supposing the patient arrests, what else can I do?' This is difficult to answer of course but if the doctor is there then external cardiac massage may permit transfer of the patient alive to hospital. The editor has seen three cases of cardiac arrest at home, each reversed by external cardiac massage and transferred to hospital alive.

Any improvement in the quality of primary care must grow from

	Patients Seen Within 2 Hours of Attack*	Patients First Seen More Than 2 Hours After Attack
Urgency	Drop everything. Go at once. (This is when patients die.)	Go as quickly as possible, but use discretion.
Care of Patient	Ease pain quickly and keep patient as still as possible.	Ease pain quickly and keep patient as still as possible.
	GIVE ENOUGH ANALGESIC TO EASE THE PAIN	Arrange treatment at home or hospital.
	Patient must remain under medical supervision for about 2 hours from onset of attack. The patient with an unstable rhythm should not be left.	Criteria are social except 1) when heart block 2) unstable rhythm
	Monitor on ECG if available.	When hospital treatment is indicated for *medical* reasons the transfer should be under a doctor's supervision.
	Do not move to hospital without a doctor preferably with monitor and defibrillator.	
	If the patient does not stabilise then transfer to hospital accompanied by a doctor.	
	If in doubt do not move the patient.	

* For the purpose of these guidelines, if there is reason to believe that a patient has had an extension of an infarction at any stage, then the risks of arrest are high and he should be treated as though he has had a second attack.

Figure 1   Summary of Guidelines

these simple facts. Doctors must examine carefully their arrangements for urgent calls. Has the practice sufficient telephone lines? Is a doctor readily available at all times? Do they need radio telephones or bleep systems? Has their staff fully understood the need for speed in these emergencies? In the early cases (less than two hours) is the doctor prepared to remain at hand until the patient is stabilised or transferred safely to hospital? These are fundamental questions which doctors must understand and answer before considering more elaborate procedures.

Drugs and Equipment

These are discussed in the following chapter.

Medical Indications for Hospital Care

In general the following may be considered as being medical indications for hospital care.

1. A patient who has suffered a cardiac arrest and been resuscitated either by external cardiac massage or defibrillator.
2. Heart block. (Although, as described by Professor Julian, many are transient and, if the patient is otherwise well, he could be managed at home. Much will depend on the particular situation.)
3. When stabilisation does not occur within a reasonable time from the onset of the attack (2-3 hours),
   (i)   Pain unrelieved
   (ii)   Ventricular tachycardia
   (iii) Runs of ventricular tachycardia
   (iv)   R on T ventricular ectopic beats
   (v)   Ventricular ectopic beats, more than 5 per minute
   (vi)   Coupling of ectopic beats
   (vii) Bradycardia
4. Other complicating medical conditions.

Shock in itself is not an indication for hospital care until better definitive treatment becomes available. Similarly, heart failure may be treated at home. If there is any doubt about moving a patient then he is probably better nursed at home.

Education

1. General Practitioners

Over the last few years general practitioners have become increasingly aware of many of the facts presented in this book. Young practitioners on vocational training courses are actively discussing and arguing about the problems of high quality primary care. However, there is little evidence that general practitioners are accepting their full responsibility and joining with hospital doctors in planning and operating community services.

2. Reception Staff

Many of the calls from patients with a myocardial infarction are placed without any degree of urgency or mention of the nature of the problem. Receptionists must be taught how to deal with calls with tact and efficiency and how to determine whether they are urgent without directly asking what the trouble is. There are few emergencies quite like this and it is the doctor's responsibility to ensure that his staff knows the common ways that patients may present.

3. The Public

The education of the public is difficult since it has its own speed of understanding. Health education may spread from the general practitioner and his team but patients will probably be influenced more by newspapers, magazine articles and television. As with doctors, it is equally important for the public to recognise that home care is appropriate in many cases but that death can sometimes occur, as indeed it may in hospital.

Importance of Records and Standardisation

The former fashions in treatment have been discussed in earlier chapters, leading up to the coronary care unit of today. We have seen how expensive care may be accepted and developed with poor evidence of its efficacy. It should be mandatory for anyone proposing a new form of care to collect data which can be assessed and compared to other treatment. It is easy to be convinced that expensive equipment with special ambulances and extra staff will achieve a greater saving of life and reduce morbidity. The community itself may be enthusiastic and encourage its doctors to provide emergency care systems. It may even donate money for equipment. However, the first generation of general-practitioner-based care services have a responsibility to prove that it is all worthwhile. The services described in Chapters 3 and 10 should be considered as experiments since they are all different and appropriate to their individual areas.

The essential information to be recorded is:

1. The age and sex structure of the population.
2. Accurate timing of events: time of onset to call; time of arrival of doctor and ambulance; time of arrival at hospital and ward.
3. Collection of electrocardiographs and serum enzymes.
4. Classification of myocardial infarction.
5. Drugs used.
6. Defibrillation.
7. Outcome at 28 days.
8. Place and time of death.

For more detailed assessment, of severity for example, then pulse, blood pressure and rhythm changes will be needed. The population being studied must be accurately defined and all deaths determined from death certificates and the coroner.

I LARGE TOWN WITH A DISTRICT GENERAL HOSPITAL WITH A CORONARY CARE UNIT AND MOBILE CORONARY CARE UNIT

Dr Brian Jones

Background

The expected incidence of acute myocardial ischaemia (including sudden death) is one or two cases per day per 100,000 population. It is likely that the time taken to reach the extremities of such a town would be in the order of from ten to thirty minutes. Since dysrhythmic death is most likely within the first hour or two the application of care to be effective would have to be within this time. The mean time of application of care ranges from 100 minutes in Belfast to 4½ hours in other units. The reasons for this delay have been discussed elsewhere.

Planning Community Care

For any attempt to shorten the delay between the onset of infarction and the application of care, it will be necessary to educate patients and those in attendance on them at home, in the factory or in the shop. In Worsley, for example, general practitioners found it difficult to do this because it was time-consuming, costly and there were ethical worries. A decision by the Local Medical Committee, the Medical Executive Committee and possibly the Area Medical Committee, would have to be made on this point. The services of the Area Medical Officer, perhaps through his Public Information Officer and Health Education Officer, should be sought.

Until recently patients have been admitted for 12-48 hours to a CCU without other consideration. However, there has been a shift in attitude with doctors looking for more specific reasons for admission, such as the presence of heart failure, dysrhythmia, unacceptable home circumstances or the fact that the incident had occurred on the factory floor, in a public place such as a place of public entertainment or a large store. If a patient had to be moved then this should be to a coronary care unit. The present attitude seems to be moving towards the monitoring of very recent cases after stabilisation, which makes movement safer within three hours from the onset. This attitude was suggested by the Mather study[2] but has been considerably influenced by the Teesside Community Survey.[3]

It follows that a mobile coronary care unit, hospital-based or community-based, is not going to influence the fatality and morbidity of acute myocardial ischaemia unless applied within the first three hours. In order to cut down on dangerous and possibly fatal delay there should be a well-publicised system for calling or summoning care. General practitioners can be equipped and organised in such a way as to share the burden of giving a coronary care service in a community and they can apply such care as effectively as a hospital-based unit. Suitable equipment, including bleep callout, has to be provided and adequate continuing training organised. This training and continuing experience should be shared with the parent coronary care unit staff at the district general hospital. It would standardise procedure, drug usage and cultivate the attitude in all concerned that this was a shared activity and not a hospital as distinct from a community activity.

At first a questionnaire could be sent to general practitioners in the district to enquire into their attitudes to coronary care and to measure their present level of activity to gain some idea of their likely cooperation. An evangelical approach on the part of the cardiologists and the more interested parties in the medical service is undoubtedly necessary not only to initiate such a service but to maintain its impetus and efficiency.

The Benefits of Group Practices or Health Centres

The structure of the general practitioner services in a district has a bearing upon the management of a community-based general practitioner coronary care service. The presence of many single-handed practitioners makes their inclusion in a rota difficult. Large groups of doctors in group practices or health centres makes it very much easier. The larger the groups and the greater the population they serve, the more experience a general practitioner member of the team would gain in the treatment of dysrhythmias. In small groups it would probably be necessary for a general practitioner to devote a period of hours only to this activity. Where there was a large grouping of doctors, other doctors of the group could excuse the duty doctor office work on his day or time on watch and he could combine this with other on-call duties.

The Future

It is considered very likely that general practitioners will take over the management of acute myocardial ischaemia along the Pantridge lines in the future but there are several factors which inhibit or prevent this at the present time. The first is that the practitioners as a body are not sufficiently well informed or persuaded of the need for or the effectiveness of intensive care. Secondly, equipment is costly and cannot be afforded; the effective use of this equipment requires training to acquire the necessary skills and efficiency and there is undoubtedly a reluctance at the present time for general practitioners to take on any additional work.

II A LARGE TOWN WITH A CORONARY CARE UNIT BUT NO MOBILE CORONARY CARE UNIT

Dr Aubrey Colling

A report of a working party of the World Health Organisation in 1974 on 'Coronary Care Outside Big Centres'[4] concluded:

> General practitioners should be made aware of the need for a quick response to calls which suggest the possibility of AMI (Acute Myocardial Infarction). A quick response means, in general, the immediate calling of an ambulance (mobile care) before trying to reach the patient personally.

Unfortunately the report gives no clear guidelines as to what a general practitioner should do if a mobile coronary care unit is unavailable, which is the situation in most areas of Great Britain.

The general principles of care described in the introduction to this chapter apply, particularly the quick response to a call, the relief of pain and remaining with the patient in the early hours after an infarction until he is stabilised. A stabilised patient is one who is free of pain with a regular pulse of normal rate. The blood pressure is of much less help in this context and rarely influences immediate future care, whether high or low.

After stabilisation, although a risk of arrest remains, it is very much reduced. If home care is undertaken then the patient should be revisited a few hours later and thereafter at the doctor's discretion. It is when stabilisation does not occur or there is a *medical* indication for hospital care that difficulty arises. There are serious risks if such patients are moved unattended to hospital. There is evidence that many die in the ambulance or before reaching the CCU in the hospital. The risks can be reduced if the doctor accompanies the patient and this is recommended. It may be necessary only once or twice a year for any doctor. He can either follow the ambulance in his car or preferably travel with the patient, an ambulance attendant following with the doctor's car. If an electrocardiograph has been used in the home, monitoring can continue en route. It may be necessary to stop the ambulance to give injections or other treatment. Speed is usually contraindicated and the general practitioner should ensure as calm and gentle a transfer as possible.

Group Care

Such arrangements are far from perfect and may soon prove unacceptable to the medical profession and the public. Groups of general practitioners may join together to form emergency care teams and there is evidence that the ethical difficulties of looking after another doctor's patients can be overcome.

III A TOWN HOSPITAL WITHOUT A CORONARY CARE UNIT

Dr Peter Berg

Although many hospitals in this country now have coronary care units (CCU), there are many areas without them where patients with proven or suspected infarcts are monitored in normal hospital wards without specialised staff in attendance. A general practitioner whose local hospital does not have a CCU must take this into account in his management of a patient with a myocardial infarction.

The First Two Hours

We have seen that about half of all deaths occur within the first two hours of the onset. If a patient is seen within this time the guidelines outlined earlier apply. In this way dysrhythmias such as bradycardia, heart block, ventricular ectopic beats, supraventricular and ventricular tachycardia can be controlled. Without special equipment, ventricular fibrillation can only be treated with external cardiac massage and hope. There is good evidence that the combined effects of the reassuring presence of a doctor, the relief of pain and the correction of dysrhythmias, as well as considerably benefiting the general condition of the patient, may also decrease the likelihood of ventricular fibrillation.

For more complete control of ventricular fibrillation a DC defibrillator is necessary. Evidence has already been given to show that this can be used by general practitioners. Defibrillators are expensive and it is likely that only specially equipped groups of general practitioners operating their own mobile coronary care unit (MCCU) will have access to this apparatus.

Further Care

At the end of two hours and when the patient has been stabilised, or when the patient is seen later than two hours after the onset, a decision must be made as to whether the patient should be kept at home or transferred to hospital. A further option may be available in certain situations, namely transfer to a distant CCU. An ordinary hospital bed may simply provide bed and board and this is all that is required for many patients. In addition to providing lodging the hospital should provide expert nursing care and close supervision of a patient with a myocardial infarct. Continuous monitoring may be available in an ordinary hospital ward during the early hours following a myocardial infarct and is a theoretical advantage of hospital admission. In this way dysrhythmias can be dealt with and ventricular fibrillation avoided.

The strains, both physical and emotional, imposed upon a close relative by looking after someone who has had a coronary must be considered. A fit, able-bodied relative is not the be-all and end-all of domiciliary care. A woman with an infarct can rarely be cared for by her working husband; indeed the anxiety arising from the consequent loss of his earnings would be likely to interfere with her recovery. Some wives may be unable to accept the responsibility of caring for a husband who may die in bed beside her. Younger patients have traditionally been treated with a period of strict bedrest followed by a programme of gradual mobilisation. Strict bedrest at home, even for washing and toilet, is very difficult to arrange and requires a particularly devoted family to achieve. More recently the period of strict bedrest has been decreased and a rather more active approach has been adopted which allows for earlier mobilisation if the myocardium is stable. In elderly patients the period of bedrest tends also to be shorter and much more emphasis is laid on progressive recovery to full activity.

Where facilities for ECG and access to biochemical investigations do not exist, or there is an unacceptable delay in obtaining the results, then hospital admission may have advantages in obtaining an earlier accurate diagnosis.

If a case of myocardial infarction is to be cared for successfully at home, by a busy general practitioner, enough time must be set aside by the doctor for adequate care at all stages during the patient's recovery, both during the initial two hours and during the time following the period of acute risk. The demands of such care have to be seen in relation to the demands of the rest of his patients and there may be times when they preclude caring for a case of myocardial infarction at home.

The potential advantages of hospital admission have to be balanced against the high mortality of patients admitted to general medical beds as shown particularly by the Teesside survey. Reports from general practice[3, 5] and the south-west study[6] have also shown that home care can provide a safe and effective alternative to hospital care in many cases. Despite this evidence a decision has to be made in relation to the specific circumstances — pathological, social, geographical and personal — of each case of myocardial infarction.

In general, if the initial consultation, within two hours of the onset of the infarct, is in the street, the surgery or the patient's place of work, then he should be admitted to hospital. These patients will require transporting and in view of the known risks of transport, it is necessary that they be moved to hospital where defibrillation is available, even within the limitations set by the absence of a CCU.

The patient's social circumstances may make hospital admission mandatory. Anyone living on their own or in poor home circumstances or in a hotel or hostel where they cannot be cared for, or where the relatives do not appear to be likely to be able to cope with the demands of home care, either for emotional or physical reasons, should be admitted.

The attitude of the patient must be taken into consideration. Many believe that hospital admission is the norm; although adequate explanation of the place of home care may overcome such attitudes, the general practitioner should not unreasonably refuse a clear request on the part of the patient or his relatives for hospital admission.

The medical indications for admission to hospital have been given earlier (see p.176). In view of the decreasing risk of death after two hours, a positive indication should be found before the patient is transferred to hospital. Admittedly there is a risk in any single individual of a late dysrhythmia which, if it had occurred in a hospital bed where a patient was being monitored, and if a suitably qualified member of the staff had seen and recognised it and was able to correct it, might not have been fatal. Such a risk has to be balanced against the unknown harmful factors in those patients who are transferred to hospital and which contribute to the hospital mortality.

Home care in the management of a patient with a myocardial infarct is more than simply caring for those who have no positive indication for hospital admission. Rather it should be considered to be the norm for the care of a patient with an infarct where the local hospital has no CCU. If the following criteria can be fulfilled home care may continue:

1. Uncomplicated myocardial infarction with stable blood pressure, normal rhythm and the absence of cardiac failure at two hours or later after the onset of symptoms.
2. Good home circumstances and supportive services.

To these may be added the need for confidence on the part of the attending physician in dealing with the risks of home care, accepting that these are no greater and probably less than those of a monitored bed in a general hospital ward.

One of the dysrhythmias which may follow myocardial infarction is bradycardia. Occasionally such a bradycardia may persist owing to a persistent A-V block. Some of these patients will require temporary pacing and a few will need to have a permanent pacemaker installed. Where a patient is found to have such a bradycardia, which persists and where a specialist cardiological unit, equipped to install a pacemaker, is within reasonable reach, it might be appropriate to transfer such a patient direct to such a unit rather than to a general hospital.

Possible Developments

Continuous monitoring is clearly necessary in the first two hours after an infarction to detect harmful dysrhythmias, but without a defibrillator all that can be done by a doctor faced with a patient who has developed ventricular fibrillation is external cardiac massage. Any improvement in the standard of primary coronary care should depend on general practitioners; on the evidence of early experiments in mobile coronary care by general practitioners, this type of approach is feasible.

Interested doctors and others within a locality could set up MCCU to care for the patients for the first two hours following the onset of an episode of infarction. At the end of this time a decision on future care would be made, if possible in consultation with the patient's own doctor. In this way the services of a fully equipped resuscitation service could be made available to all patients within a locality without the implication that all patients with infarcts will be admitted to hospital. Such a service would be generally beyond the means of a single group practice. It should cover a limited geographical area, covering a population of 40,000 to 70,000 to allow for easy and rapid access to the patient without overloading the service. The equipment required is fairly expensive but, by setting geographical limits, appeals for funds could be made to the community within the area. Previous experience shows that the necessary funds can usually be raised without too much difficulty.

Other problems would need to be overcome; for example the way in which patients are referred to the service, the natural reluctance of some general practitioners to have other doctors involved in the primary care of their patients, the reluctance of the public to call early in the presence of suspicious symptoms and the release of general practitioners from their routine work. Such a scheme would require the active cooperation of the ambulance services and local hospitals.

Any doctor who has experienced the sense of helplessness when faced with a patient with ventricular fibrillation will recognise the value of a MCCU which could be based on general practice.

IV   A SMALL COUNTRY TOWN WITH A COTTAGE HOSPITAL

Dr Brian Sproule

A cottage hospital is an ideal centre for primary care equipment in the form of mobile packs. These packs should be easily identifiable and kept together in a room so that a doctor going to a suspected case of myocardial infarction can pick them up easily and quickly or delegate someone else to do this for him. It is necessary for the monitor and defibrillator to be kept on constant trickle charge prior to being taken.

A member of the nursing staff of the cottage hospital should be made responsible for the supervision of the equipment and replenishing drugs and appliances when used or as they become out of date. Ideally the nurse responsible should have had training in coronary care so that she can train the other nurses in the cottage hospital in the use of primary care equipment for the immediate treatment following an infarction, including cardiac resuscitation. The nurses would then be available for any ambulant case of myocardial infarction coming into the cottage hospital unexpectedly prior to the arrival of a doctor. They would also be able to accompany cases in ambulances if they are transferred to a coronary care unit.

Doctors attached to the cottage hospital might find it suitable to work in groups so that one of them could be on immediate call in rotation and available to go at once to any suspected case of myocardial infarction. It is not thought advisable that he should have the equipment in his car all the time as the monitor and defibrillator could not then be charged, and breakages may occur in the case containing the drugs which could lead to a serious shortage at a vital time. There should be some arrangement whereby the primary care equipment can be taken to the doctor in the district if by chance he encounters a myocardial infarction unexpectedly. Ideally the duty doctor should be in radio telephone communication to ensure his accessibility.

A cottage hospital can be considered as a convenient extension of home treatment, in that transferral of a case to it involves minimal disturbance of the patient's environment and ensures easy access for his close relatives. In many cases, therefore, where home treatment is impossible the cottage hospital will be the next best thing. When considering transfer further afield to either a general medical ward or a coronary care unit, this must receive very careful thought, particularly where the ambulance journey involved will take longer than thirty minutes. At the present time not enough is known of the reasons why a patient's prognosis is worsened by an ambulance journey of over thirty minutes,[7] and the advantages of admission to a coronary care unit may be outweighed by the hazards of the journey. It should be noted, however, that cottage hospitals are not suitable for prolonged monitoring of cases and it is justifiable to withdraw monitoring after a period of three hours from the onset of an infarction. The occurrence of ventricular fibrillation is very much reduced after this time but of course it can still occur. However, the advent of drugs to prevent prophylactically the onset of ventricular dysrhythmias will lessen the risk in the future.[8]

V   A COUNTRY PRACTICE WITHOUT A COTTAGE HOSPITAL

Dr Robert Pawson

If the essence of primary coronary care is the speed of arrival of informed medical aid then this is the rural practitioner's major problem. Most surveys have shown the long delay in calling the doctor's surgery. This is more evident in rural areas with the different attitudes of these patients to illness. The next delay is in contacting the doctor who is often working on his own in a large and sometimes inaccessible area. The third delay is the time taken to reach the patient's home, sometimes prolonged for reasons of terrain and travelling distance. The decision about hospital admission is also affected by the same factors in relation to location of patients to surgery, coronary care unit and ambulance base. Means to improve these problems are essential for satisfactory coronary care. (Radios are not the complete answer as geographical conditions frequently make communications unreliable.)

Single-handed practitioners should group together to form rotas for coronary care and, where geographical conditions allow, existing small group practices could enlarge by further grouping to make more economical use of time and equipment. The equipment itself will often affect the size of groups since it must be suitably located for all participating doctors, to reduce the delay in obtaining it. The equipment could be kept at a central surgery where a doctor or his messenger could collect it, or at the local ambulance base. It must be the aim in organising groups in rural practice to ensure total cooperation of all colleagues as numbers are inevitably small.

The basic principles for deciding which patient to admit to a coronary care unit are little different from any other type of practice but special factors will modify these principles. Some patients prefer home care whilst patients living alone are less likely to obtain the necessary support from relatives to allow home care to continue.

Any defibrillated cases should be admitted, similarly uncontrolled dysrhythmias and all cases of heart block which do not readily come under control. (Even uncomplicated cases of first degree block if the patient lives in an outlying area or one with difficult access.) Complicating medical or nursing problems should also indicate admission. Availability of nursing staff may add to the difficulties in isolated areas with only one 'triple-hatted' nurse. (Health visitor, nurse and midwife.)

Once admission has been decided upon the doctor should accompany the patient, continuing to monitor rhythm and rate to ensure the most safe and comfortable journey to hospital. The problem of returning to the practice from the coronary care unit will require local solution. The other problem of covering the single-handed doctor's duties would be solved by 'rota' formation or by using techniques developed when domiciliary midwifery was the vogue.

Special equipment (i.e. non-personal) includes the monitor/ defibrillator, oxygen and intravenous infusion sets. This poses problems for every type of practice as regards cost but in rural practice the cost per doctor will be greater due to lack of numbers, which is further reduced by geographical problems limiting its own efficiency. An ECG machine may be included in this list for similar reasons. Without such equipment a comprehensive policy of care is not possible as we now know that a significant percentage of early deaths are a consequence of ventricular fibrillation and the Oxford study[7] showed that increased distance from hospital increased the need for DC shock therapy. Long ambulance journeys increase the problems of monitoring machine reliability. This suggests that a monitor would be superior to attempting the same technique with an ECG machine. However, with these aids and intensive care, speed of admission becomes a secondary factor.

These facts, however, should not preclude rural practitioners from setting up a primary care service as in a large number of cases stabilisation of the patient's condition prior to removal to the coronary care unit is possible with ECG monitoring and a knowledge of drugs in common use. Rural practice poses no special problems with drug therapy apart from the possibility that time intervals until admission, including ambulance journey, may necessitate greater total doses of antidysrhythmic therapy than usually suggested in previous reports. Records are important in rural practice, particularly where there are various people involved in the care of one patient. Education of the community may pose more problems in rural areas. Urgent requests for the doctor which involve admission to hospital are often automatically linked with the non-return of the patient from hospital.[9] Rural populations are less inclined to follow urban trends that associate 'proper care' with hospital admission. Thus pressure to admit in doubtful cases is not so evident and may be opposed where long distances are involved. It has been shown that education of a rural community is possible to some extent through personal contact with patients, local organisations and specially organised meetings.[10]

Notes

1. Pantridge, J.F., 'Mobile Coronary Care', *Chest,* 1970, 58, 229.
2. Mather, H.G. *et al.,* 'Acute Myocardial Infarction: Home and Hospital Treatment', *British Medical Journal,* 1971, 3, 334-8.
3. Colling, W.A. *et al.,* 'Teesside Coronary Survey: An Epidemiological Study of Acute Attacks of Myocardial Infarction in a Large Urban Community', *British Medical Journal,* 1976, 2, 1169-72.
4. World Health Organisation, 'Coronary Care Outside Big Centres', Report on a Working Group. Copenhagen, 4-5 November 1974.
5. Sleet, R.A., 'Report of 24 Cases of Myocardial Infarction Treated at Home', *British Medical Journal,* 1968, 4, 675-7.
6. Mather, H.G. *et al.,* 'Myocardial Infarction. A Comparison between Home and Hospital Care for Patients', *British Medical Journal,* 1976, 1, 925-9.
7. Acheson, R.M. and Sanderson, C., 'Myocardial Infarction: Home and Hospital Treatment', *British Medical Journal,* 1976, 2, 105.
8. Zainal, N. *et al.,* 'Disopyramide in the Treatment and Prevention of Arrhythmias following Myocardial Infarction', *Journal of International Medical Research,* 1976, 4 Supplement (1) 71.
9. Personal observation.
10. B. Sproule, personal observation.

12 DRUGS AND EQUIPMENT

Dr Aubrey Colling

Drugs

A general practitioner needs a limited number of drugs for the primary care of patients after myocardial infarction. He will use analgesia in every case, other drugs less commonly. Since he may only require drugs other than analgesics once or twice a year, it may be advisable to carry them in a separate box together with makers' instructions and contraindications or other guidelines.

The following notes may be of help:

Pain

Pain must be completely relieved and it is important to give sufficient analgesia. The first dose should be given intravenously, repeated in 10-15 minutes, either intravenously or intramuscularly, if pain is still present Diamorphine (heroin) 5 mg or morphine 15 mg.

Diamorphine is less likely to have cardiovascular side effects. Both drugs may be combined with cyclizine (Valoid) 50 mg or prochlorperazine mesylate (Stemetil) 12.5 mg to reduce vomiting. Freeze-dried diamorphine should be used.

Entonox (50 per cent nitrous oxide, 50 per cent oxygen) gives effective relief of severe pain and is often available in ambulances. For later control of pain, tablets such as dipipadone hydrochlor (Diconal) or suppositories, for example oxycodone pectinate (Proladone) 30 mg are useful.

Bradycardia (< 55/min.)

Bradycardia should be treated with aliquots of intravenous Atropine 0.6 mg, usually only when there are complications, for example, hypotension and dysrhythmias. Atropine clears rapidly from the blood (2-4 hours) and the dose may need to be repeated several times to achieve benefit. It can also improve partial heart block.

Tachycardia (> 120/min.)

If no electrocardiograph is available to ascertain the nature of the tachycardia, it is safe to use Practolol.

Supraventricular Give practolol in 5 mg aliquots intravenously. It may take twenty minutes to work. It is contraindicated in asthma and obstructive airways disease and should be used with extreme caution in heart failure.

Ventricular Lignocaine in 50 mg aliquots intravenously given over 1-2 minutes. (Lasts 10-20 minutes.) Also when ventricular ectopic beats ($> 5/$min.), coupling of ventricular ectopic beats, runs of ventricular tachycardia, multifocal ectopics and R on T ectopics. Lignocaine intravenously may be followed by an intramuscular injection of 300 mg if a patient is being transferred to hospital.

Heart Failure

Digoxin and diurectics (e.g. frusemide (Lasix) 40 mg) may be necessary but not usually in the very early hours after an attack.

Other less commonly used drugs which should be carried: Heparin and Warfarin for anticoagulation; Isoprenalin Sulphate for heart block (if symptoms warrant it) and cardiogenic shock.

Equipment

Several intravenous injections may be necessary and it is useful to introduce a Butterfly or Venflon Cannula at the beginning of care. They are available with different sized needles.

At the National Workshop on Coronary Care held in Cleveland in 1976, a number of firms exhibited equipment of value to general practitioners who might be introducing intensive care to their primary care team. The electrocardiograph should now be considered an essential tool for any general practitioner, not only for treating myocardial infarction but for the investigation of chest pain, dysrhythmias and hypertension. On the other hand, defibrillators are relatively expensive and will be used very rarely by an individual practitioner unless he is part of a large team geared to intensive care and very early call. Money for such equipment is unlikely to be forthcoming from official sources and it would be a good opportunity for the community to contribute by voluntary subscription, a pattern emerging from schemes already operating. It is recommended that general practitioners who contemplate buying such equipment should visit the schemes already operating. In general, equipment should be lightweight, easy to use and reliable. The general practitioner will probably be on his own and though the equipment seen in coronary care units may be very elegant it may be more complicated and heavier than necessary.

British Oxygen Comapny Limited

Entonox (50 per cent nitrous oxide, 50 per cent oxygen) is useful for pain relief and is supplied either from patient demand equipment or by continuous flow measurement. (In a double blind trial it was shown[1, 2] that severe cardiac pain was relieved effectively after myocardial infarction, though not when pain was only moderate or slight. After 10 minutes use this benefit could no longer be demonstrated when compared to a control group. Entonox therefore might be of value when a patient's pain has not been relieved and he is being transferred to hospital.) Elizabeth Way, Harlow, Essex CM19 5AB. (Tel: 0279 29692)

Cambridge Medical Instruments

The Transrite 5 electrocardiograph (fig. 1) is mains powered and has mains rechargeable cells for dry batteries. It does not conform to the American Heart Association recommendations for specifications for

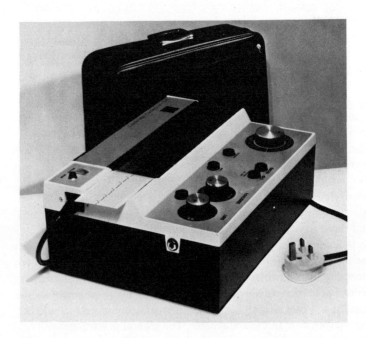

Figure 1   The Transrite 5

instruments used in electrocardiography but such high standards are not required for use in general practice. The VS4 model reaches these standards but it is more expensive. The Transrite 5 is a well developed and widely used machine. Weight: 15 lb + 7½ lb for the carrying case and accessories. The company also makes a variety of monitoring equipment. Melbourn, Royston, Herts. SG8 6EJ. (Tel: 0763 60611)

Cardiac Recorders Limited

The Electrocardiograph made by this British company, the Minigraph 123 (Figure 2) is mains operated with internal rechargeable batteries. The recording is made on paper using a thermo-chemical reaction which is less easily damaged than the wax paper widely used. (Weight, including accessories, 15½ lb.) This firm also sells the Pantridge mini-defibrillator with rechargeable batteries, weighing only 7.7 lb and a miniature monitor (Type 290) weighing only about 1 Kg. 34 Scarborough Road, London. N4 4LU. (Tel: 01-272 9212)

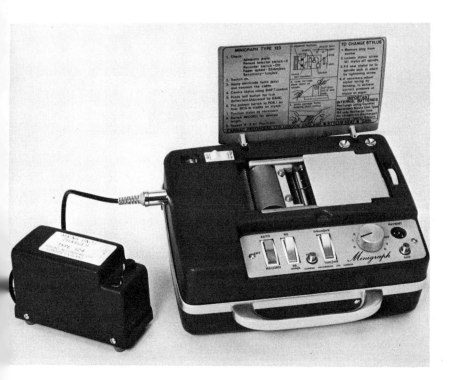

Figure 2 The Minigraph 123

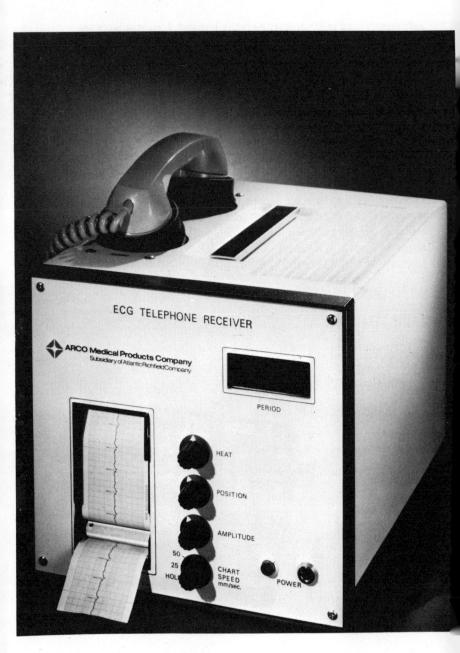

Figure 3   The Arco Receiver

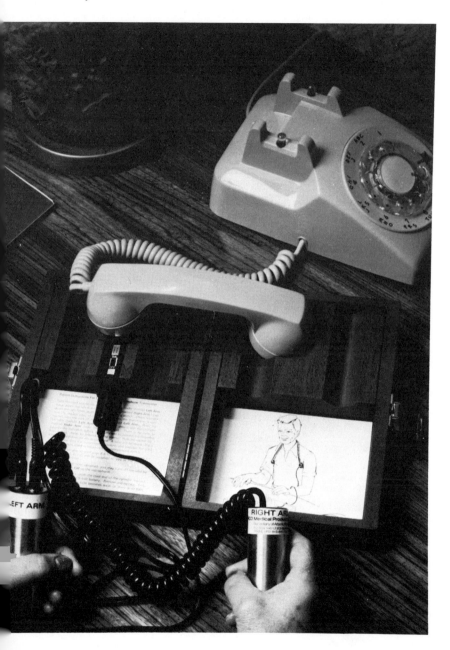

Figure 4   The Arco Transmitter

Charles F. Thackeray Limited

This company distributes the Arco ECG telephone receiver. (Figures 3 and 4). Two electrodes are held by the patient and the cardiograph is transferred by telephone to a hospital or other centre. P.O. Box 171, Park Street, Leeds. LS1 1RQ. (Tel: 0532 42321)

Linton Instrumentation

The Viscard 8 (Figure 5), distributed by this company, is a miniature cardioscope which, in an emergency, can be pressed directly on to a patient's chest without any leads or cables. For monitoring, a power supply can be used and electrodes attached in the conventional way. (Weight 4.5 lb.) Hysol, Harlow, Essex. (Tel: 0279 24606)

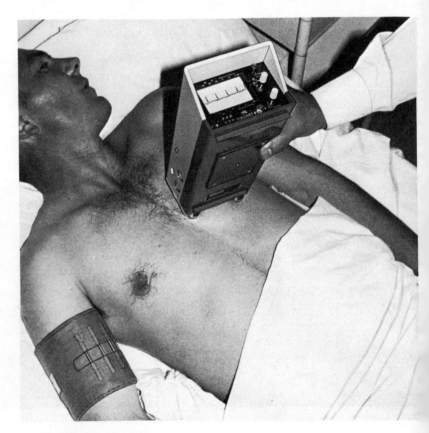

Figure 5   The Viscard 8

Simonsen and Weel Limited

The Cardio-aid (DMS 200) (Figure 6) is a battery operated monitor defibrillator with a memory cardioscope and synchronised defibrillation. (Weight 34 lb.) Hatherley House, Hatherley Road, Sidcup, Kent. DA14 4BL. (Tel: 01 300 1128)

Vitalograph

This firm deals largely with respiratory instruments. The complete intubation, resuscitation and aspiration set (specification 24000) contains a hand-powered resuscitator of the self-filling bag type. (Weight 7½ lb.) Maids Moreton House, Buckingham. MK18 1SW. (Tel: 02 802 3691)

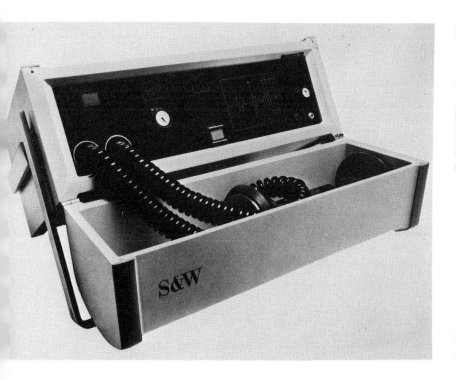

Figure 6   The Cardio-aid (DMS 200)

Notes

1. Kerr, F. *et al.*, 'Nitrous-Oxide Analgesia in Myocardial Infarction', *Lancet,* 1972, 1, 63.
2. Kerr, F. *et al.*, 'A Double-Blind Trial of Patient Controlled Nitrous-Oxide/ Oxygen Analgesia in Myocardial Infarction', *Lancet,* 1975, 1, 1397.

PART FOUR   REHABILITATION AND
PREVENTION IN GENERAL PRACTICE

13 THE REHABILITATION OF THE CORONARY PATIENT

Dr Aubrey Colling

A recent Royal College of Physicians report[1] states that 'those who care for patients with heart attacks should have rehabilitation in mind from the very beginning'. Though this is an admirable concept, a more definitive approach with clear guidelines is needed to avoid unnecessary invalidism. It is now better known that though physical incapacity may follow a myocardial infarction, it is equally common for psychological and social factors to be the cause of failure to resume a normal life and return to work.

It is also becoming clear that the general practitioner has an important role in coordinating the rehabilitation of patients. In those cases he keeps at home, he will assume full responsibility from the beginning and ensure that he undertakes the two interviews (or two series of interviews) which are described later. He will also complete the investigation of patients for risk factors and set them on an optimistic course to full physical and mental conditioning. The difficulties are greater when patients have been treated in hospital. Firstly, because of the division of responsibility amongst hospital doctors, advice to patients may be sketchy and poorly understood by them. A brief chat on a ward round and the distribution of a rehabilitation booklet by the sister or houseman is no substitute for a one-to-one discussion. To be effective, this may need to be repeated several times by the same doctor. When the patient returns home the general practitioner must at once determine not just what his patient has been told, but what he understands. He will then be in a position to formulate a plan for his rehabilitation.

Though hospital rehabilitation can be very good, there is evidence that many patients are badly informed and do not have a clear idea of what has happened to them, and what can be expected of them in the future. Similar comments can no doubt be applied to some home treated cases, but in the Teesside survey, criticisms were nearly all from patients who had been treated in hospital. Typical notes made by the survey nurses were:

Feels very strongly that he was kept in the dark.

The patient was entirely unaware that he had had a heart attack.
The patient felt that he had not been able to rest enough whilst in
    hospital.
The patient said that he was not really told anything.
Claims that he was told in hospital that he would have another
    infarction and feels that he is 'under sentence of death'.
Told that he had heart trouble but nothing was explained to him
    at all.
Anxious, and expressed resentment towards the hospital.
Not satisfied with GP's care — he feels his doctor does not take
    enough time to talk to him or listen to his complaints.

Complaints were equally divided between those directed against the
hospital and those expressing lack of continuity on the part of their
general practitioner after discharge from hospital. However, there was
no doubt in the minds of the nurses undertaking the interviews, that
those patients who had been kept at home had a far better grasp of
what was going on and a greater appreciation of the more positive
aspects of rehabilitation.

Though these remarks are critical, there were others which
expressed satisfaction with what was done for them in hospital and
for the way their general practitioner looked after them, either at
home or on return from hospital. For example:

Very pleased with treatment.
Has been closely followed up by his general practitioner, and has
    been well informed about his illness.
Satisfied with his GP.
The GP discussed with him very fully about his illness.
Very happy with the care he received in hospital.
Feels that he is well informed about his illness.

Similar remarks were given to Mayou and his colleagues who
interviewed forty patients and their relatives after a myocardial
infarction in Oxford.[2]

Patients found it difficult to recall the early stages of illness. At the
initial interview most were satisfied and indeed very grateful for the
quality of their care, in both the coronary care unit and the general
wards, but seemed to have very little understanding of diagnosis,
the nature of hospital treatment, or longer term implications.

When interviewed after discharge patients still seemed to have very little understanding of the possible implications of their illness and recalled very little medical advice.

A further difficulty in hospital-treated cases is that patients frequently return home taking a variety of tablets — diuretics, beta blockers, iron, hypnotics and vitamin C. Most general practitioners are reluctant to stop these drugs which are usually unnecessary. The result is that many patients continue to take drugs long after an infarction, without good reason, and at a time when a more active, health-orientated rehabilitation should be planned. Such continued drug taking focuses attention on treatment and disease rather than on health and trying to alter a faulty life-style. Though certain drugs, such as clofibrate (Atromid) or beta blockers, may offer a theoretical advantage, a more healthy attitude might be engendered in patients if all drugs were avoided in uncomplicated cases and attention paid to other aspects of rehabilitation.

Similarly, the follow-up of patients by hospitals should be discouraged unless a carefully planned rehabilitation service is offered or there is a special medical indication. A casual follow-up appointment two or three months after an attack may even delay a patient's natural desire to return to work.

Teesside Rehabilitation Survey

The Teesside Coronary Survey, described in Chapter 3, included a rehabilitation study which illustrates some of the factors involved and is of particular value in being a community study, including both home and hospital cases.

There were 219 male patients under sixty-five years of age who had been working at the time of the onset of the attack and who survived. Information was obtained on 185 of these patients, 26 by postal questionnaire and 159 by interview. Twenty per cent were home-treated and 80 per cent hospital treated.

Return to Work

From national sickness benefit statistics, it is known that about half the patients return to work within ninety days of their attack but there can be considerable delay in the remainder. In an investigation in Birmingham[3] it was found that about half the patients who had not resumed work had no signs of cardiac damage or failure and that anxiety and depression were very common. Others had been advised or influenced not to return to work by their doctors or friends. Where rehabilitation is actively pursued, as in a Dublin experiment, a much higher return to work rate can be achieved when compared to patients not receiving the benefits of such adivce.[4]

In the Teesside Coronary Survey 60 per cent of the men who had a definite myocardial infarction returned to work within three months. There was no detailed assessment of why the others had not returned though most of them gave the reason that their doctors still regarded them as unfit. In only one case did a patient say his doctor considered him to be fit, while he did not.

Of those back at work, 82 per cent had not changed their job, the remainder were doing work of a lighter nature. Most men had returned without restrictions of any kind.

Health Factors

No special attempts were made by the survey team to influence patients' behaviour other than the general advice given to patients at the time of the study. Fifty-three per cent claimed to have lost weight deliberately though nearly a quarter had actually gained weight. Twenty-seven per cent of the smokers claimed to have stopped and many of the others had cut down significantly. About a third, however, had not changed their habits and 4 per cent had actually increased. Almost two thirds of patients were attempting to restrict their diet in some way.

Twenty-Eight-Day Visit

As part of the survey, many of the patients were visited after twenty-eight days by the survey nurses for a further electrocardiograph and assessment. Patients seemed to welcome these visits and were eager to talk to them about their illness and the future. The survey was designed to observe behaviour rather than to influence patients so that no formal medical or rehabilitation advice was given.

The main impression gained by the survey nurses was of the great uncertainty in patients' minds at the time of this visit. Specifically, many patients said that they were not sure of the diagnosis or what had happened to them. They did not know how much they were allowed to do nor when they would be able to return to full activity. They were also in the dark about what could or should be done to prevent a recurrence.

Most of the deficiencies lay in the poor communication between patient and doctor, and between hospital physician and general practitioner. Nor was it known when patients were most likely to understand and retain what was discussed with them, or indeed how often they needed to be told.

The Role of the General Practitioner

There are two important interviews which must be undertaken by the general practitioner. They can only be considered to have been completely successful when the general practitioner is sure that his patient has understood what has been discussed, and this may take several consultations.

1. The first interview begins soon after the attack, as soon as the patient is free of pain and the acute phase is over. Though a brief explanation may have been offered at the height of the attack, there comes the moment, usually after 36-72 hours, when the question is asked, 'What has really been the matter, doctor?' This is the opportunity to sit down and explain frankly to the patient what has happened and what can be expected of him in the future. Though this interview is described in terms of men because the condition is commoner in men than in women, there is the same need for rehabilitation in women. The doctor should always be optimistic and say that he expects him to return to full activity (which is nearly always possible), that he will be able to return to full employment without any restrictions (which is usual), and that he will be encouraged to take more physical activity than he did before (which is often advisable).

   Following this, the cautious rehabilitation of the next few weeks is described. If the patient makes no such enquiries within three days then the doctor should take the initiative.
2. The second interview takes place at about two or three weeks after the attack. If the first phase has been successful the patient should now be eager to be more active. Full conditioning should now begin, aiming at complete functional recovery 8-12 weeks from the attack so that work can be resumed. The nature of the patient's work and his physical condition will determine the exact length of convalescence.

   More important, the future will be discussed, again in optimistic terms. After return to work he will be expected to increase his activity even further; to swim, walk, cycle, run or whatever activity he finds most appealing. The various risk factors will be discussed; the sad fact is that they will usually have been present for twenty years or more, patients having disregarded the advice of doctors or what they know to be true from their own common sense. At this emotional time they may now heed advice.

The interview is best conducted in the presence of the spouse. If the patient has been treated in hospital then it should begin at the first visit after discharge. The husband is usually the first in the family to have had a myocardial infarction but the risk factors, such as faulty eating habits, inactivity and cigarette smoking, may be common to all family members. The interview should be considered to be a family one and a general change in life-style may be recommended.

At some stage the patient will wish to resume car driving, gardening and sexual intercourse. After the first few weeks such activities can be gradually restarted. It has been estimated, for example, that the energy cost of sexual intercourse is roughly equivalent to brisk walking or climbing 1-2 flights of stairs.[5] Such facts should be introduced in this interview.

Estimation of serum lipids should be made about two months after the attack but nothing should delay the conditioning programme already under way. If a well-defined optimistic programme is planned from the outset then few of the difficulties described later will develop.

For those who are older or have a poorly functioning myocardium then less ambitious programmes should be planned. However, the doctor should not be misled by the apparent severity of the initial attack into believing that an excellent recovery is impossible or unlikely. Perhaps, in the past, this danger has not been fully recognised and doctors and patients have both tacitly accepted the inevitability of ill health and restrictions after a heart attack.

Early Identification of Patients with Risk of Poor Rehabilitation

Though optimism should prevail throughout rehabilitation, it must be acknowledged that some patients will fail to make a good recovery. Cardiac damage and non-cardiac psychological and social factors have been found to be equally common causes of failure.[3] When medical factors are of prime importance, physical conditioning may be an advantage, though it is often ineffective or even contraindicated.[6, 7] When cardiovascular recovery has been good then successful rehabilitation mainly depends on psychological and social factors.

Dr Cay and her colleagues studied the rehabilitation of 203 male patients in an Edinburgh coronary care unit,[6, 7] and they were able to identify those who were likely to have difficulties.

Age

Old patients do better than young ones; particularly prone are those aged 35-44.

Social Class

Professional and managerial classes are least likely to have problems.

Severity of Attack

Severity plays only a small part in delaying rehabilitation except in those who retire prematurely.

Immediate Emotional Upset

Those who have an immediate and severe emotional reaction to their heart attack may well be depressed and anxious some months later.

Patient's Personality

Those who have coped well in the past with other problems of adult life adjust successfully. Those who have reacted in the past with neurotic disturbance are likely to have considerable difficulties.

With care it may be possible to recognise patients at risk and avert invalidism. Facilities for late rehabilitation are described in detail in the report of a Joint Working Party of the Royal College of Physicians of London and the British Cardiac Society. ([1] Table p.299)

Physical Conditioning

Even though they may be desirable, there are only a handful of units in Britain able to offer physical testing or retraining after myocardial infarction. Nevertheless, the underlying principles, which have recently been reviewed[1] are of considerable help to the practising physician.

Response to Physical Conditioning

Patients respond to physical conditioning in the same way as healthy subjects of comparable age. The benefit is in the improvement to the oxygen transport system which is believed to occur in the peripheral circulation and muscles rather than in the heart itself. Whether there is an associated improvement in myocardial perfusion and contractility is uncertain. The response to physical conditioning depends on the intensity, duration and frequency of exercise. The effects are summarised summarised in Table 1.

Table 1: The Effects of Physical Training*

Regular physical activity has been shown to:

Increase	Decrease	
Maximum oxygen intake	Arterial systolic pressure)	
Work performance	Heart rate)	at any given
Maximum cardiac output	Ventilation)	oxygen intake
Mitochondrial enzyme activity in skeletal muscle	Blood lactate)	
	Myocardial oxygen uptake)	
Joint mobility and skeletal muscle strength	Obesity	
	Convalescent depression	

and may

Increase	Decrease
Safety of vigorous exertion	Risk of sudden death
Coronary collateral circulation	Catecholamine production
Physical coordination and dexterity	Serum triglycerides
	Vulnerability to dysrhythmias
	Blood coagulation
	Convalescent postural hypotension
	Insomnia

---

*From the Report of the Joint Working Party of the Royal College of Physicians of London and the British Cardiac Society on Rehabilitation after Cardiac Illness.[1]

Degree of Expected Improvement

The increase in maximum oxygen intake obtainable by physical training is between 7 per cent and 33 per cent and work that was previously difficult can then be performed with relative ease. There is also an additional improvement (5 per cent to 7 per cent) in mechanical efficiency. If these can be achieved by exercise which is enjoyable and suits the tastes of the patient then so much the better.

Patients who are limited by angina derive most benefit. In an investigation by Bruce[8] the maximum oxygen intake increased by 10 per cent in a healthy group of men, 17 per cent in a post-infarction group and 42 per cent in a group of patients with angina. Well-designed trials have shown that patients who exercise after an infarction not only have an enhanced capacity for work but gain a morale boosting effect from their training.[10, 11]

Type of Exercise

Formal exercise in a gymnasium is not everyone's idea of fun, yet some patients undoubtedly benefit from such group activity. Others may prefer walking, cycling, swimming or golf.

There should be graded increase in work during training, each phase lasting seven to ten days. The general practitioner should review the patient as he thinks appropriate. Exercise should be taken regularly, at least twice, and preferably thrice, weekly. To be effective it requires, eventually, a degree of vigour producing at least slight dyspnoea and sweating.

Heavy isometric exercise (such as prolonged press-ups and carrying weights) is generally believed to be unsuitable since it overloads the left ventricle. For details of exercise tests and conditioning reference can be made to special studies.[1, 9]

Notes

1. 'Report of Joint Working Party of the Royal College of Physicians of London and the British Cardiac Society on Rehabilitation after Cardiac Illness', *Journal of the Royal College of Physicians of London,* 1975, vol.9, No.4.
2. Mayou, R., Williamson, B., Foster, A., 'Attitudes and Advice after Myocardial Infarction', *British Medical Journal,* 1976, 1, 1577-9.
3. Nagle, R., Gangola, R., Picton-Robinson, I., 'Factors Influencing Return to Work after Myocardial Infarction', *Lancet,* 28 August 1971, 2, pp.454-6.
4. Mulcahy, R. and Hickey, N., 'The Rehabilitation of Patients with Coronary Heart Disease', *Journal of the Irish Medical Association,* 1971, vol.64, no.422, 541-5.
5. Hellerstein, H.K. and Friedman, E.H., 'Sexual Activity and the Post-Coronary Patient', *Archives of Internal Medicine,* 1970, 125, 987.
6. Cay, E.L. *et al.,* 'Return to Work after a Heart Attack', *Journal of Psychosomatic Research,* 1973, 17, 231-43.
7. Cay, E.L., Vetter, N.J. and Philips, A.E., 'Practical Aspects of Cardiac Rehabilitation: Psycho-Social Factors', *Giornale Italiano di Cardiologia,* 1973, vol.III, no.5, 646-55.
8. Bruce, R.A., 'Is Physical Training Beneficial in Patients with Coronary Heart Disease?', *Controversies in Medicine,* 1973, vol.II.
9. 'Myocardial Infarction. How to Prevent and Rehabilitate', sponsored by the Council on Rehabilitation, International Society of Cardiology. 1973. (Printed by Boehringer Mannheim)
10. Sanne, H., 'Exercise Tolerance and Physical Training of Non-Selected Patients after Myocardial Infarction', *Acta Medica Scandinavica,* 1973, supplement 551.
11. Kentala, E., 'Physical Fitness and Feasibility of Physical Rehabilitation after Myocardial Infarction in Men of Working Age', Thesis. University of Helsinki, 1972.

14 THE PREVENTION OF CORONARY THROMBOSIS

Dr Aubrey Colling

Today, general practitioners and hospital physicians believe they are in the front line dealing with an epidemic affecting nearly everyone in so-called Western society and killing one in two of those who have a heart attack; not unnaturally they are preoccupied with treatment. Nevertheless, doctors should pay some attention to the causes of the disease to determine whether they have a part to play in prevention. A recent report of a Joint Working Party of the Royal College of Physicians of London and the British Cardiac Society[1] says,

> The prevention of CHD (Coronary Heart Disease) in the community is predominantly the role of the general practitioner and the Working Party considers that the continuation and extension of good general practice should provide the main means of identifying high risk subjects.

The Working Party, however, does not recommend mass screening but rather 'Selective Health Examinations' of those especially at risk. How realistic is this approach? Would it be likely to alter the epidemic materially? Is it right that the general practitioner should shoulder such a responsibility? Such a question is asked because during a time of diminishing resources we must look carefully at the effectiveness of care and put weight behind those measures which are most likely to succeed.

Is Myocardial Infarction a Preventable Disease?

First of all, is myocardial infarction a preventable disease? There seems to be general agreement that it is environmental in origin. As previously discussed it was first fully described earlier this century[2, 3] and there is no convincing evidence that it was common but unrecognised in former days. Osler and MacKenzie are said to have recognised very few cases though in a careful review in 1967 Robb-Smith[4] stated: 'There is no known evidence for an increased age specific incidence of coronary thrombosis or myocardial infarction from English or American post-mortem studies.' He attributed the apparent increase to different classifications of disease, a changing pattern of post-mortem techniques and to an altered age structure of cases examined. Despite this evidence clinicians and epidemiologists appear to accept that there has been a true increase in the illness they recognise as 'Acute Myocardial Infarction' (AMI), even though coronary artery atheroma must have been present in earlier days. Since 1950, though there have been some changes in the classification of ischaemic heart disease, it has been possible to compare yearly fatality rates and an increasing incidence has been observed in many countries.[5]

There is now considerable evidence that the illness occurs rarely or never in many communities but that when people move from an area of low incidence to an area of high incidence, they soon develop the high incidence of their adopted country.[6] For example, it has been shown to occur in Japanese and Africans who in general have a low incidence of AMI and who take on the disease pattern of North America when they move there. Moreover, African and European children in South Africa are born alike with regard to their blood chemistry but by the age of seven the European children have increased blood fats.[7]

It would be an attractive solution to find a single cause for AMI yet all that clinicians and epidemiologists have discovered are a series of associated or risk factors. Critics point out that the cause of tuberculosis was also considered to be multifactorial until the causative organism was isolated.

Nevertheless, other factors such as housing, nutrition and working conditions played a part in that epidemic which was causing more than 10 per cent of all deaths (including infants) at the end of the Victorian era.[8]

What Are the Possible Causes?

'Western' Diseases

It is necessary to discuss possible causes of AMI prior to embarking on preventive measures in general practice though it is inappropriate to do this in detail in a work of this kind. It is worth stressing that AMI is only one of many diseases with a high prevalence in developed countries such as appendicitis, peptic ulcer, gall stones, obesity, varicose veins, dental caries, diverticular disease, bowel cancer and diabetes. Burkitt[9] has pointed out that environmental factors must be primarily responsible for all these diseases since they are often found together and the order in which the frequency of each arises in different communities following the adoption of a Western pattern of life, appears to be relatively constant. Taylor,[10] for example, has described the experience of Dr Paddon in Labrador after the Eskimos came into contact with civilisation. First came sugar and dental caries, cigarettes followed and within ten years three new diseases made their appearance — coronary artery disease, peptic ulcer and chronic bronchitis.

Such changes have long been recognised. In a book which has become a classic, Weston Price, an American dentist in the years before the Second World War, visited various communities throughout the world, some of which were still living primitively while others had only recently become Westernised.[11] He described people in the isolated Swiss valley of Loetschental and the Isle of Lewis in the Hebrides as well as Eskimos, North American Indians and Africans. Everywhere the story was the same. The 'simple' native diets protected the teeth, modern diets quickly caused decay and led to deformed crowded teeth with changed facial appearance in later generations. He was impressed by the general health of native people. By contrast he claimed that in North America those states which had been longest occupied by modern civilisation had the highest mortality levels from heart disease. Moreover, he believed in the value of milk products of high quality and analysed many thousands of butter samples. He produced yearly graphs showing that the mortality of heart disease followed inversely the curve of vegetation growth.

In a well-known series of experiments performed more than forty years ago, Sir Robert McCarrison[12] compared the poor diet of the Southern Indian to the better diet of Indians in the North. Those in the South had many nutritional deficiencies and when he fed their diet to rats they did less well than rats fed the better diet of Northern Indians. Now, Dr Malhotra, the Chief Medical Officer of the South Eastern Railway in India, has reported coronary artery disease to be fifteen times less common among North Indian railroad sweepers aged eighteen to fifty-five, even though they consumed 11 per cent more fats from milk and fermented milk products compared with South Indian railroad sweepers in the same age group. Moreover, the Southerners ate little fat and what they did consume was from unsaturated fatty acids of seed oils.[13]

More recently Dr Crawford, of the Nuffield Institute of Comparative Medicine in London, has examined the diets and state of health of several African peoples and has made inferences with regard to coronary artery disease.[7] He warned of the dangers of monocultures and also searched for the harmful effects of changes in the diets of animals. He described the work of Dr Laws on elephants in Uganda. In certain areas of the National Parks a combination of man-made fires and elephant activity had in a short space of time destroyed the Terminalia woodland, leaving only scrubland grass. The stomach contents of normal elephants consist largely of woodland products; the stomachs of these Uganda elephants contained 95 per cent grass. The elephant food structure had been changed from a fibrous oil-rich natural diet to the soft, water-rich products of the grassland. Fertility declined and infant mortality increased. Because of this evidence elephants were culled and one of the most striking findings on post-mortem examination was gross arterial degeneration not dissimilar to that seen in humans. Elephants of the same age living more naturally in forest showed no evidence of gross arterial damage.

Fats and Carbohydrates

Dr Crawford also stressed the importance of structural fat and criticised previous writers who had not distinguished clearly between structural (invisible) fat and adipose tissue (visible fat). The building blocks of fat are the fatty acids. Two essential fatty acids are Linolenic Acid (from greens, bark and leaves) and Linoleic Acid (from seeds, nuts and berries). They cannot be synthesised by animals or man though they are necessary for growth and development. Man can gain his supply directly from whole grain, green vegetables, nuts and berries or indirectly from animals and fish. Structural fats in the body are associated with protein and contain a diversity of fatty acids, saturated, mono-unsaturated and polyunsaturated. By contrast adipose tissue is contained in fat cells and consists largely of triglycerides from non-essential saturated fatty acids.

Cholesterol has been much studied in relation to ischaemic heart disease, perhaps because it was one of the first substances in plasma to become readily measured. Though it is a precursor of steroid hormones and bile salts and is present in cell membranes its biological importance is poorly understood. Dietary cholesterol is only responsible for 10 per cent to 20 per cent of the body pool, the remainder being synthesised, largely by the liver. Cholesterol synthesis and the enterohepatic circulation of bile acids form a vital homeostatic mechanism controlling the level of cholesterol in plasma and the body pools. The amount of cholesterol absorbed may be influenced by dietary fibre. Plasma cholesterol levels are known to relate closely to the risk of developing AMI but since the synthesis of cholesterol involves some of the products of carbohydrate and triglyceride metabolism it is difficult to know how important dietary cholesterol is.

In our preoccupation with cholesterol and coronary artery disease we appear to have ignored the importance of structural fat in our diet. The wild animals around us on which we feed do not appear to carry adipose tissue to any great extent and the fat from venison, hares, rabbits, fish and other free-range animals is rich in polyunsaturates. Excess saturated fat can displace structural fat in the body and comes either directly from the fat which is eaten or from the conversion of sugar in the liver. There has been much debate between the 'sugar' and 'fat' schools of thought in the aetiology of AMI but it would seem that the two are closely related.

The intake of sucrose has increased several times since 1850.[6] In times of poverty and hunger all sugar is utilised for energy. Howe[8] quotes an Inter-departmental Committee Report in 1904 which found that 33 per cent of all children were undernourished and hungry. (Twelve-year-old public school boys were five inches taller than those from council schools!) In times like these, for most people there would be little sugar left for conversion to fat. Storage fat which consists largely of triglycerides is the body's main store of energy. Fat consumption also rose and presumably was metabolised by people short of calories for energy. In recent times, however, there has been an excess of both fat and sugar in our diets and if saturated lipids are important factors in coronary artery disease it is easy to understand how such a surplus could arise.

In a most remarkable book, *The Saccharine Disease*, Dr Cleave[14] focused attention on the increase in sugar consumption over the last 150 years and the low levels of fibre in our refined carbohydrate diet. He attributes a wide range of environmental diseases to this deficiency, from acute appendicitis and varicose veins to diverticulitis and coronary thrombosis. Unfortunately he did not distinguish between structural and adipose fats in his arguments. Nevertheless, in a foreword, Dr Burkitt endorses the opinion of Sir Richard Doll on the predictions of Cleave and his colleague Dr Campbell and the likelihood of them proving correct, 'if only a small part of them do, the authors will have made a bigger contribution to medicine than most university departments or medical research units make in the course of a generation'.

A man of 52, a patient of the author who had a severe infarction, appeared at first sight to have none of the recognised risk factors. However, he worked in a sugar factory and was found to consume large quantities of sugar and had Type IV lipoproteinaemia.

Other Risk Factors

Other so-called risk factors are better understood by doctors. Cigarette smoking, obesity, hypertension, softness of water and lack of physical activity are all associated with an increased frequency of myocardial infarction though they are not causal. The contraceptive pill also carries a threefold increase in risk in women over forty. The increased risk with the male sex is great and of considerable academic interest. All these risk factors are additive and the evidence is neatly summarised in the Joint Working Party Report.[1]

An ingenious method of summating these risks has been devised by Dr Khosla and his colleagues.[15] Using established data on American and European men aged between forty and fifty-nine they calculated the relative risk for four factors, age, cholesterol level, systolic blood pressure and number of cigarettes smoked. The relative risk for each factor is obtained from tables and multiplied to give a 'risk predictor' figure. The result can then be compared to the range of risk run by 1,000 men of a given age.

The Package

How then can the general practitioner play his part in prevention? From what has been said it is clear that he probably has an impossible task. Impossible that is, to influence the national statistics on incidence. Yet he has a duty to his patient and must be able to give advice when it is required and this may often be in a preventive capacity. Specialist advice such as referred to earlier[1, 6] is too restrictive for the general practitioner who, because of his wider role, will not wish to confine himself to coronary artery disease alone. Much is unknown about environmental diseases of this kind but it is becoming clear that a wide knowledge of several disciplines is required in order to understand and influence what we see. For want of a better word I will call this 'the Package'.

Infant Feeding

Let us begin with birth. Though most doctors pay lip service to breast feeding they have not improved the low national incidence of breast feeding. Very few know the hazards of cows' milk (artificial feeding) as summarised in recent publications.[16, 17] Turner has pleaded that 'Breast is best for coronary protection'.[18] When doctors are asked how strongly they try to persuade mothers to breast feed they concede that they never exert undue pressure on them. Compare this to the way many doctors insist on the treatment of hypertension. Yet there is evidence, from post-mortem studies of babies and young people who had died inadvertently and who had been bottle fed, that they had changes already present in their arteries.[19] These changes ranged from an accumulation of muco polysaccharides to fully developed atherosclerotic plaques. Offering babies cows' milk is common in many midwifery units in the first few days despite the dangers of introducing foreign protein during that time.[20] A leading article in the British Medical Journal claimed: 'Formula feeding carries the double risk not only of depriving the infant of IgA but at the same time of exposing it to potent immunogens in cows' milk itself.'[21]

Sugar too is often fed with water. Every farmer knows the importance of feeding newly born animals directly from the mother in the first few days of life and the difficulties that arise if this is unsuccessful. The immunological and other responses of animals and man are different but when so much is unknown it must surely be wise to insist on breast feeding whenever possible.

Antenatal Care

But even before birth we are neglectful. Cigarette smoking in mothers is known to produce smaller babies. If it is a risk factor for adult arterial disease then surely it must be bad for the arteries of babies? Doctors have a captive population attending at regular intervals for antenatal examinations but how many women receive guidance about smoking or other nutritional matters? The growing foetus especially needs structural fat. Do we ensure it gets sufficient? Discussing breast feeding opens up many possibilities for prevention.

Already then during the process of birth we see the need, in the prevention of coronary artery disease, for doctors to have some knowledge of nutrition, human and animal behaviour and immunology. We do not know how important all this is in the prevention of coronary artery disease but, though certain proof is lacking, there is strong circumstantial evidence of its value, alongside its other proven advantages. We can begin to see some of the deficiencies of medical education which by being so disease-orientated has failed to prepare us for preventive work. As Dr Crawford has pointed out, 'Every medical school has its department of pharmacology but there is only one teaching department of nutrition in Britain.'

Quality of Food

Though we pay little attention to what our patients eat, we are even less interested in the quality of their food and know next to nothing of how it is produced. We are preoccupied with obesity and the quantity they consume. A leading article in the *British Medical Journal*[22] asked, 'Are polyunsaturated fatty acids harmful?' and concluded: 'It is disturbing that we consume commercially processed foods without considering what they contain, how they are made or what harm they may do.'

It is only fair to point out that a group of doctors in Cheshire played a part in the formation of the Soil Association many years ago to promote proper care of the soil and to encourage organic farming.[23] Few doctors understand farming and are not greatly interested in the way their patients' food is produced. For example, beef as supplied to the public varies from one part of the country to another. The beef in Glasgow contains a much higher percentage of fat than that sold in the South-east of England. Even within the city of Glasgow the fatter and cheaper portions of the carcass tend to be sold in the poorer areas of the city.[24] This kind of information may be important in helping to explain the high incidence of AMI in North-west Scotland.

Social History

We also need to have a knowledge of history and the ecology of people as described so delightfully by a geographer, Professor Howe.[8] For example, there is a considerable regional variation in the household consumption of certain foods. There is a higher than average consumption of cakes and biscuits in Scotland together with a lower intake of fresh green vegetables; the reverse is true of South-east England. Changes in smoking habits show that at the beginning of the century only 12 per cent of tobacco consumed was in the form of cigarettes. In Professor Howe's *Atlas of Disease Mortality*[25] the incidence of coronary artery disease is shown region by region and can be compared with other diseases.[10] In a similar way Drummond and Wilbraham's *History of the Englishman's Food*[26] describes the changing patterns of our diet. It is only when we look at the way our present food is grown that one doubts whether the composition of butter, milk and meat as well as vegetables is similar now to former times, or even to other parts of the world.

Anthropology

Even an understanding of anthropology is of help. It has been widely
assumed that man was essentially a hunter and gatherer in evolutionary
terms. Ardrey, in *The Hunting Hypothesis*[27] questions this and believes
we killed to live. Gathering was not our main source of food in the days
before fire which occupied most of our evolutionary history. Recent
analysis of human 'coprolites' (which are dessicated or petrified remains
of faeces) shows that no plant remains are being found in the very early
specimens. By contrast remains of plant fibres and seeds are found in
old American Indian deposits which are of more recent origin. Settled
agriculture is very recent and is believed only to go back ten thousand
years.

It would appear that those who advocate certain cereal diets or the
restriction of animal products in the prevention of coronary artery
disease have much explaining to do.

Agriculture

The nutritional aspects of coronary artery disease are extremely
complex. So much so that official committees in Britain can only
agree on a formula of a reduction of sugar and fat in our diet, together
with keeping down patients' weight. (The recommendations in other
countries are summarised by Ball and Turner.)[28] Common sense would
seem to dictate that more should be done. There is little mention of
agriculture yet many of our policies are difficult to follow in health
terms. Our stock animals are fattened on grain which we can ill afford.
The customer in any case does not want the fat which may be harmful
to him, the butcher can not sell it yet farm prices and subsidies are
often based on such fattening. Food subsidies themselves often seem
inappropriate – as in the case of subsidies for butter and bread, for
example. It is difficult to see how the general practitioner can influence
such policy changes. Dr Turner of the Department of Preventive
Cardiology in Edinburgh has begun to investigate this area of concern
and has found that farmers would be willing to change their present
practices if different national policies could be agreed.[24]

Risk Factors

Can the doctor influence the recognised risk factors associated with
coronary artery disease – smoking, hypertension, obesity,
hyperlipidaemia and alck of exercise? There are certainly many
opportunities in the everyday work of a general practitioner to detect

those at risk from the environmental diseases of Western society, for example, the many obese patients who attend our surgeries, those complaining of a variety of bowel complaints such as people with peptic ulcer and constipation, and those with frequent respiratory infections. There is a whole range of conditions which can alert the doctor to such problems. Indeed the main difficulty in prevention is not recognition but whether a doctor is prepared to spend time on health education and whether patients and families will accept his advice and change their behaviour. Unfortunately, human behaviour being what it is, most of us are not prepared to alter our life-style until after a crisis such as AMI has occurred.

Secondary prevention is applied by most doctors to the survivors of attacks of myocardial infarction though we do not know how effective it is either in general or in the long term. Certainly patients are then more receptive to advice. There is experimental evidence in animals that arterial changes are slowly reversible and other reports suggest that regression has occurred in human beings both in war time and in people with infection or cancer.[29] It is worth stressing yet again that secondary prevention for the first affected family member, usually the husband, becomes primary prevention for the remainder — a potential field for health education. The increased risk in women over forty taking the contraceptive pill should be remembered.[30]

Whether regular screening should be undertaken as advocated by some,[31] or selective health examinations are recommended by the Joint Working Party,[1] is questionable. Indeed the latter recommendation is a curious one since it presupposes a prior general screening to identify those who need the selective health examination. Most other screening procedures have yielded disappointing results and new ones should only be considered on an experimental basis at the present time. Dr Rankin is at present conducting a feasibility study in an Edinburgh general practice. In a preliminary report[32] he showed that 106 (57 per cent) of a group of men aged between thirty-five and forty-four accepted an invitation to participate and that eighty-nine were seen a second time between six and twelve months later. Personal details were obtained by a health visitor at a home visit followed by specific advice on diet, smoking and exercise. A subsequent examination by the general practitioner included height, weight, skin fold thickness, blood pressure, urine, ECG and chest X-ray. At follow-up there was evidence of improvement in weight, lipids and smoking habits similar to that found by others, for example, Stamler[33] in Chicago. The cost of this programme has been seriously underestimated, however, and if applied generally would be prohibitive. Nevertheless, several experiments of this kind should be supported to find out how effective they would be.

In a specialised book such as this it is tempting to be enthusiastic about prevention but one must remember that the general practitioner is responsible for a wide range of disease and disorder. I find it difficult to support the formal conclusion of the Working Party which advocated selective health examinations. In answer to the questions posed earlier, 'Is it likely that selective health examinations would alter the epidemic nationally?' and 'Is it right that the general practitioner should shoulder such a responsibility?', I think we must say no. The screening of say 100 patients per general practitioner per year might cost the health services between £50 million and £100 million per year. No one can advocate such expenditure without careful consideration. There may be better ways of practising prevention and giving health education. Other forms of research, together with government legislation and changes in agricultural policies may well prove more effective in the long run.

The general practitioner might be better advised to study further the subjects briefly discussed in 'the Package' in order to become more conscious of the processes of health. Such knowledge will influence his everyday work and perhaps have a wider effect than health examinations restricted to coronary artery disease.

Notes

1. 'Prevention of Coronary Heart Disease', Report of a Joint Working Party of the Royal College of Physicians of London and the British Cardiac Society, *Journal of the Royal College of Physicians,* 1976, vol.10, no.3.
2. Obratzow, W.P. and Straschesko, N.C., 'Zur Kenntnis Der Thrombose Der Koronarterien Des Herzens', *Z. Klin. Med.,* 1910, 71, 116.
3. Herrick, J.B., 'Clinical Features of Sudden Obstruction of the Coronary Arteries', *Journal of the American Medical Association,* 1912, 59, 2015.
4. Robb-Smith, A.H.T., *The Enigma of Coronary Heart Disease,* London, 1967.
5. Epstein, F.H. and Krueger, D.E., 'The Changing Incidence of Coronary Heart Disease', in *Modern Trends in Cardiology,* Chapter 2, London, 1969.
6. Department of Health and Social Security, *Diet and Coronary Heart Disease,* HMSO, London, 1974.
7. Crawford, M. and S., *What We Eat Today,* London, 1972.
8. Howe, G.M., *Man, Environment and Disease in Britain,* New York, 1972.
9. Burkitt, D.P., 'Some Diseases Characteristic of Modern Western Civilisation', *British Medical Journal,* 1973, 1, 274.
10. Taylor, Lord, 'Poverty, Wealth and Health, Or Getting the Dosage Right', *British Medical Journal,* 1975, 2, 207.
11. Price, W.A., *Nutrition and Physical Degeneration,* California, 1945.

12. McCarrison, R. and Sinclair, H.M., *Nutrition and Health,* London, 1953.
13. Malhotra, S.L., 'Protective Role of Dietary Factors in Coronary Heart Disease', *Practitioner,* 1976, 217, 929.
14. Cleave, T.L., *The Saccharine Disease,* Bristol, 1974.
15. Khosla, T., Newcombe, R.G. and Campbell, H., 'Who Is at Risk of a Coronary?', *British Medical Journal,* 1977, 1, 341.
16. 'Present-Day Practice in Infant Feeding', Report of a Working Party of the Panel of Child Nutrition, Committee on Medical Aspects of Food Policy, Department of Health and Social Security, HMSO, London, 1974.
17. Davies, P.A., 'Feeding', *British Medical Journal,* 1971, 2, 351.
18. Turner, R.W.D., 'Breast Is Best for Coronary Protection', *Lancet,* 1976, 2, 693.
19. Osborne, G.R., *Incubation Period of Coronary Thrombosis,* London, 1963.
20. Gerrard, J.W., 'Breast Feeding: Second Thoughts', *Paediatrics,* 1974, 54, 757.
21. 'Breast Feeding: The Immunological Argument', Leading Article, *British Medical Journal,* 1976, 2, 1167.
22. 'Are PUFA Harmful?', Leading Article, *British Medical Journal,* 1973, 4, 1.
23. 'Nutrition, Soil Fertility and the National Health', Cheshire Panel Committee Supplement to the *British Medical Journal,* 15 April 1939, p.157.
24. Turner, R., personal communication, 1976.
25. Howe, G.M., *A National Atlas of Disease Mortality In The United Kingdom,* London, 1963 (2nd revised and enlarged ed., 1970).
26. Drummond, J.C. and Wilbraham, A., *The Englishman's Food,* London, 1939 (new, rev. ed., 1957).
27. Ardrey, R., *The Hunting Hypothesis,* London, 1976.
28. Ball, K.P. and Turner, R., 'Realism in the Prevention of Coronary Heart Disease', *Preventive Medicine,* 1975, 4, 390.
29. 'Regression of Atherosclerosis', Annotation, *Lancet,* 1976, 2, 614.
30. Mann, J.I., Inman, W.H. and Thorogood, M., 'Oral Contraception Use in Older Women and Fatal Myocardial Infarction', *British Medical Journal,* 1976, 2, 445.
31. Turner, R. and Ball, K., 'Prevention of Coronary Heart Disease: A Counterblast to Present Inactivity', *Lancet,* 1973, 2, 1137.
32. Rankin, H.W.S. *et al.,* 'The Control of Coronary Heart Disease Risk Factors in General Practice: A Feasibility Study', *Health Bulletin,* May 1976.
33. Stamler, J., 'Prevention of Atherosclerotic Coronary Heart Disease', in *Modern Trends in Cardiology,* chapter 6, London, 1969.

CONTRIBUTORS

Professor Roy Acheson, M.A., D.M., F.R.C.P., F.F.C.M., Professor of Community Medicine University of Cambridge.

Dr Jennifer Adgey, M.D., M.R.C.P., F.A.C.C. Consultant Physician, Royal Victoria Infirmary, Belfast.

Dr Peter Berg, BM BCh., D.Obst. R.C.O.G., General Practitioner, Broxbourne, Hertfordshire.

Dr Douglas Black, M.D., Medical Superintendent, Baie Verte Peninsula Health Centre, Newfoundland.

Dr Douglas Chamberlain, M.D., F.R.C.P., Consultant Physician, Royal Sussex County Hospital, Brighton.

Dr Aubrey Colling, M.D., F.R.C.G.P., General Practitioner, Stockton-on-Tees, Cleveland.

Dr Clifford Cowley, M.A., D.C.H., D.A., D.Obst.R.C.O.G., General Practitioner, Ramsey, Isle of Man.

Dr Alex Dellipiani, M.D., F.R.C.P., Consultant Physician, North Tees General Hospital, Stockton-on-Tees, Cleveland.

Dr David Hill, MB BS., M.R.C.P., Lecturer in Medicine, University of Nottingham.

Professor Desmond Julian, M.A., M.D., F.R.C.P., F.R.A.C.P., Professor of Cardiology, University of Newcastle-upon-Tyne.

Dr Brian Jones, MB ChB., General Practitioner, Worsley, Manchester.

Dr Robert Mayes, MB BS., Medical Officer, Imperial Chemical Industries, Billingham, Cleveland.

Dr Robert Pawson, MB ChB., D.Obst.R.C.O.G., M.R.C.G.P., General Practitioner, Great Ayton, North Yorkshire.

Dr Brian Sproule, MB ChB., M.R.C.G.P., General Practitioner, Coldstream, Berwickshire.

INDEX

bsasa2 g

hypotension 113

incidence of attack 20, 86; and social
    class 64, 65; by age 40-2; by
    population 42, 77-8, 178; by sex
    40-2; in Brighton 133
incidence of premonitory symptoms
    44-6, 47
incidence of ventricular fibrillation
    101
India, diet in 210
industrial medical department 143-6
    staff 143
infant feeding 213-14
infusion techniques 131
intensive care 94
intubation techniques 131
isoprenalin sulphate 191

lectures 131
lignocaine 93, 117-19, 131, 136,
    157, 191
linoleic acid 211
linolenic acid 211
Linton Instrumentation 196

McCarrison, Sir Robert 210
metoclopramide monohydrochloride
    (Maxolon) 111
mode of onset 51
monitoring 98-100, 116, 134, 140,
    152, 160-1
mortality 94; and social class 65;
    causes 53
mortality rate 183; by sex 51
morphia 109, 111
morphine 89, 190

nitrous oxide 89
Norris index 52
notification 50, 85, 133, 158;
    delays in 84, 87, 94-5;
    improving 179; procedures 39.
nurses 186
nutrition 214-16

oscilloscopes 134
oxycodone pectinate (Proladone)
    190
oxygen-giving equipment 162, 197

pacing 91, 184
pain 95-6, 109, 111-12, 174, 190-1;
    effects 89; relief of 88-9
Pantridge, Prof. J. F. 107, 130

Pantridge defibrillator 151, 193
parasympathetic overactivity 104-5
Parker, Dr. William 130, 132
patients: and changes in life-style
    202; and follow-up interviews
    203-4; and physical conditioning
    205-7; and twenty-eight day
    visit 202-3; attitudes of 183;
    chances of return to work 27;
    complaints 199-200; risks in
    moving 18, 32, 160, 166, 181,
    183, 186; satisfaction with
    treatment 200-1; time off work
    201-2; with poor rehabilitation
    risk 204-5
Peel index 28, 52, 55-6, 59
pethidine 89, 111
physical conditioning 205-7
place of care, selection of 85
population density, effect on journey
    time 34
Practolol 113, 116, 190
'pre-infarction syndrome' 44
premonitory symptoms 44-6, 47
Price, Weston (dentist) 210
primary care 107, 109, 111, 113-26,
    134, 152-3, 164-7, 180; by rural
    practitioner 187-8; delays in
    administering 94-5, 95-6, 100,
    109; formulating policy for 173-4,
    175; improving quality 174-5,
    184-5; in absence of mobile
    unit 180-1; in first two hours
    181-2; need for haste 26; *see also*
    care after stabilisation
primary care case 161, 168, *see also*
    equipment
primary research team 38
prochlorperazine mesylate 190
Proladone 190

radio 151
radiotelephones 156, 175
Ramsey group practice 155-9
records 153, 161, 177-8, 188
rehabilitation 199-207; and drug-
    taking 201; Teesside survey
    of 201-3
resusication, results of attempted
    138-9
risk factors 213
road system 34
Robb-Smith, A.H.T. 208
Royal College of Physicians 199;
    Joint Working Party of RCP and